THE
HAPPY
GUT
GUIDE

THE HAPPY GUT GUIDE

Copyright © Summersdale Publishers, 2018

Text by Wendy Green

An Hachette UK Company
www.hachette.co.uk

Vie Books, an imprint of Summersdale Publishers Ltd
Part of Octopus Publishing Group Limited
Carmelite House
50 Victoria Embankment
LONDON
EC4Y 0DZ
UK

www.summersdale.com

Printed and bound by CPI Group (UK) Ltd, Croydon, CR0 4YY

ISBN: 978-1-78685-245-8

Substantial discounts on bulk quantities of Summersdale books are available to corporations, professional associations and other organisations. For details contact general enquiries: telephone: +44 (0) 1243 771107 or email: enquiries@summersdale.com.

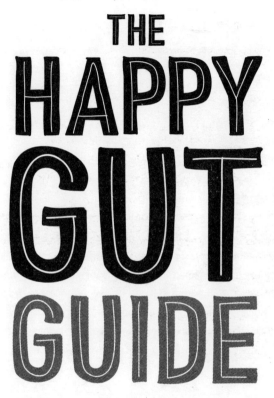

THE HAPPY GUT GUIDE

KNOW MORE, LIVE WELL, FEEL GREAT

WENDY GREEN

Disclaimer

Every effort has been made to ensure that the information in this book is accurate and current at the time of publication. The author and the publisher cannot accept responsibility for any misuse or misunderstanding of any information contained herein, or any loss, damage or injury, be it health, financial or otherwise, suffered by any individual or group acting upon or relying on information contained herein. None of the opinions or suggestions in this book is intended to replace medical opinion. If you have concerns about your health, please seek professional advice.

CONTENTS

Introduction – The Glorious Gut...**7**

Part 1: The Grumpy Gut...**15**
Chapter 1 – Signs and Causes of an Unhealthy Gut....................**16**

Part 2: Food and the Gut...**29**
Chapter 2 – Fill Up on Fibre...**30**
Chapter 3 – Get to Grips with Gluten...**34**
Chapter 4 – Sugar – Not So Sweet...**39**
Chapter 5 – Heal Your Gut with Healthy Fats............................**50**
Chapter 6 – Why Your Gut Needs Protein.................................**54**

Part 3: Balance Your Biome...**59**
Chapter 7 – Eat Your Gut Happy...**60**
Chapter 8 – Sleep Your Gut Healthy...**90**
Chapter 9 – Dial Down Stress...**99**
Chapter 10 – Get Gut Active...**116**

Part 4: A Gut-Loving Day...**123**
Chapter 11 – Breakfast...**124**
Chapter 12 – Lunch...**133**
Chapter 13 – Dinner...**143**
Chapter 14 – Fermented Pickles and Gut-Friendly Dips............**155**

Final Thoughts..**163**

Jargon Buster...**164**

Resources...**168**

Products...**170**

Acknowledgements..**172**

About the Author...**173**

INTRODUCTION

THE GLORIOUS GUT

Most people think of the gut simply as the part of our body that digests the food we eat. But exciting new research now shows that it has a much wider role in our physical and mental well-being, and it may all be down to the tiny bacteria that live there.

The gut hosts over 100 trillion bacteria collectively known as the microbiome, which outnumber the cells in your whole body. These tiny microbes work very hard for us in exchange for us giving them an environment where they can flourish. They turn undigested food into various hormones, enzymes, chemicals and vitamins that influence our weight, digestion, mood, general well-being and even how much pain we feel. They also protect us from foreign invaders, and have a huge role in our immune system. Our individual mix of gut bacteria makes each of us the unique person we are. In this book you'll learn how changing your microbiome can change not just your health but also your life and find lots of advice and tips to help you do just that.

Where did my gut bacteria come from?

When you were in the womb your gut would have been sterile. If you had a normal birth and were breastfed you would have picked up some beneficial bacteria such as *Bifidobacteria* and *Lactobacilli* from your mother, which not only protected your health then but also formed the basis of your future well-being. You would have also picked up bacteria from your birth surroundings and the people around you. On the other hand, if you were born by caesarean and bottle fed, your gut may have been colonised by less beneficial bugs. A lack of 'good' bacteria in your gut in the first year is linked to a bigger risk of suffering from allergies, gluten intolerance and weight gain in later life.

Your microbiome would have grown and multiplied for the next three to five years until it was similar to an adult's in terms of its composition and diversity. Over the course of your life you will have continued to pick up bacteria from other people and your surroundings – both indoors and outdoors. These bacteria will have grown and multiplied massively – the average adult has trillions of bacteria in their intestines from over 400 different species.

'Good' and 'bad' bacteria

The gut microbiome contains both beneficial ('good') and hostile ('bad') bacteria. To have a healthy microbiome you need to have more good than bad bacteria.

What else affects my gut bacteria?

Other influences on the type of bacteria you have in your gut throughout your life include the types of foods you eat and how often you take antibiotics. Antibiotics don't just kill off bad bacteria but also good ones. Stress and lack of sleep, as well as gut infections and food poisoning, can also affect the balance of the microbiome by encouraging the growth of bad bacteria, as we will see in **Chapter 1**. There's also evidence that smoking reduces the number of healthy bugs in the gut and damages the gut lining too. Levels of friendly flora in the gut also tend to decline as we age, making us more prone to tummy bugs. When the healthy balance between good and bad gut bacteria is out of kilter it's known as dysbiosis, which is linked to digestive problems like wind, bloating, indigestion and irritable bowel syndrome (IBS). It's also associated with more serious health problems which we'll look at in **Chapter 1**.

The 'gut-brain'

When we talk about having a 'gut feeling' or 'gut instinct' we are not far wrong – the gut contains the same types of nerves and cells found in the brain. A network of over 100 million nerves, known as the enteric system, extends from our throat to our bottom. Often referred to as the 'gut-brain' or 'second brain', the enteric system connects the gut to the brain, enabling them to exchange messages. This helps explain why some of us lose our appetite, or even suffer from tummy ache, when we are upset or worried.

What exactly is the gut?

The gut is another name for the digestive system (or tract) which is about 9 m long and includes the mouth, oesophagus (food pipe or gullet), stomach, small intestine, large intestine (colon or large bowel), rectum (back passage) and anus (bottom). These hollow organs are lined with mucous membranes known as mucosa, or gut lining. The mucosa in the mouth, stomach and small intestine has tiny glands that release juices to help digestion. Inside the gut there is also a layer of smooth muscle that contracts to help break down food and push it along. This is called peristalsis.

Did you know?

Your gut lining is only one cell thick, which means it's far thinner than your eyelid and can easily be damaged. It replaces itself every three days.

How does the gut digest food?

Digestion involves mixing food and drink with digestive juices, pushing them along the gut and breaking them down into the smallest possible pieces, so that they can be absorbed into the bloodstream through the walls of the intestines. It begins in your mouth and ends at your bottom. Now let's take a brief tour of the key organs involved in digesting your food.

The mouth and teeth

When you chew your food, you break it down into smaller pieces and mix it with saliva. Saliva contains an enzyme called amylase, which starts breaking down carbohydrates (starch) into sugars.

The oesophagus

Swallowing food triggers peristalsis, which forces it down your oesophagus through a muscular valve known as the lower oesophageal sphincter (LOS), into your stomach. This valve stops food and stomach acid coming back up your gullet.

The stomach

Once in the stomach, food is mixed with gastric juice, which contains the enzymes protease (pepsin) to break down protein and lipase to digest fats, and hydrochloric acid which kills most of the bacteria (good and bad) in the food. The resulting thick liquid is called chyme. The mucosa in your stomach produces mucus to protect its lining from the acid and protease, and to help lubricate the food to make it easier to push along the gut. An average meal usually takes about 4 hours to empty from the stomach and pass into the duodenum.

The small intestine (duodenum, jejunum and ileum)

The chyme travels down to the duodenum, which is the first part of your small intestine. The small intestine, at around 6 m long, is actually the longest section of the gut and is where 90 per cent of food digestion and absorption takes place. In the duodenum, bile from the liver neutralises acids and dissolves fats in the partially digested food. This allows enzymes in the pancreatic juices to further break down carbohydrates and proteins, and start digesting fats. This semi-liquid then passes into the second part of the small intestine – the jejunum.

The jejunum releases more of the enzymes that break down carbohydrates into glucose (sugar), proteins into amino acids and fats into fatty acids and glycerol, which are then absorbed into the bloodstream and carried around the body. The remaining digested food particles then travel into the last part of the small intestine, the ileum, where vitamin B12 is absorbed and bile salts are reabsorbed. This process takes the small intestine around 2–6 hours depending on the types of food you've eaten. Beneficial *Lactobacilli* tend to live in this part of the small intestine, where they feed off the food particles, making enzymes such as lactase and folic acid (a B vitamin) and lowering blood cholesterol.

The large intestine (colon)

Unabsorbed food matter then travels into the large intestine (colon), which is shorter and fatter than the small intestine. Here other bacteria such as *Bifidobacteria* and *Escherichia coli* feed off it, breaking it down (fermenting it) still further and making important minerals like magnesium and calcium easier to absorb. During this process they produce short-chain fatty acids, B vitamins needed for energy and good mental health, and vitamin K for blood clotting. These vitamins, and water, are absorbed in the large intestine.

Helpful bacteria also prevent the more harmful strains from multiplying by using up oxygen and nutrients. They play an important role in helping us to digest our food and obtain as many nutrients as possible from it. Meanwhile, the gut provides a safe place for them to live – making it a mutually beneficial relationship.

Undigested insoluble fibre, bacteria, dead skin cells from the digestive tract lining, proteins, fats and water form faeces (poo) that are stored in the rectum before being passed out through the anus.

How long does it take to digest a meal?

The average length of time it takes for food to pass through the digestive system is about 18 hours, depending on how fast the muscles contract and the type of food eaten. Sugars and refined carbohydrates are digested the quickest. Proteins, fats and fibre take much longer to be absorbed, so they keep you feeling full for longer, which is helpful if you want to lose weight.

Digestive helper organs

The pancreas, liver and gall bladder are often referred to as the digestive 'helper' organs, as they play an important role in digestion. The pancreas produces a juice that contains enzymes that break down protein, fat and carbohydrates. It also releases the hormone insulin, which enables the body to use sugars. The liver filters blood from the gut, stores nutrients and produces bile. The gall bladder stores bile and releases it into the small intestine after a meal to help digest fat.

You now have a basic understanding of your gut and the huge role it plays not only in your digestion, but in your overall well-being. Read on to find out how you can maximise your health by making your gut happy with the right diet and lifestyle choices.

Part One looks at the causes of an unhealthy gut, including a poor diet, certain medications, insufficient sleep, a lack of exercise and excessive stress. It explains how eating too many sugary and processed foods and not enough fruit, vegetables and wholegrains (prebiotics) and fermented foods (probiotics) encourages an overgrowth of 'bad' gut bacteria which are linked with type 2 diabetes and digestive, immune, weight, mental health and skin problems. You'll also learn about the symptoms of other gut-related health issues like ulcerative colitis and Crohn's disease and when to seek medical advice.

Part Two explores how your gut handles the different components of food including fibre, gluten, sugars, fats and protein foods such as meat, and the effects they can have on your gut and general health. You'll also discover the signs and causes of gluten sensitivity and coeliac disease, as well as fructose and lactose intolerance.

Part Three gives you the low-down on the diet and lifestyle choices that will balance your microbiome and make your gut happy. You'll find out which foods and drinks can help boost your friendly flora and how eating mindfully can improve your digestion and help you avoid overeating and problems like wind and bloating. There are also tips to help you de-stress and sleep better, which will help soothe your gut. As exercise also helps to improve gut health, you'll find easy ways to sneak more physical activity into your daily life too. You'll also discover how a happy gut means a healthier you.

Part Four outlines a gut-loving day. Here you'll find easy-to-follow gut-friendly diet tips, including foods to try and foods to avoid. You'll also find delicious beneficial-bug-boosting recipes, including how to make your own probiotic yogurt and pickles.

This is followed by a **Jargon Buster** that explains the meaning of the gut-related terms with which you may be unfamiliar.

Finally, the **Resources** section lists a selection of books, websites and products you may find helpful.

PART 1

THE GRUMPY GUT

CHAPTER 1

SIGNS AND CAUSES OF AN UNHEALTHY GUT

Like any other part of the body, things can sometimes go wrong with the gut. In this chapter you'll find an overview of common digestive problems that can arise when the balance between good and bad gut bacteria is out of kilter – such as bloating, constipation and IBS. The gut plays a major role in our immune system. So it follows that if the healthy balance between good and bad microbes is disrupted, the immune system can react inappropriately. This can cause inflammation and autoimmune disorders like ulcerative colitis and Crohn's disease. Other signs of an unhealthy gut – such as weight gain, skin problems, diabetes and low mood – and when you should seek medical advice are also covered in this chapter.

Bloating and wind

Bloating can be due to excess wind, often caused by eating too fast or eating when you are feeling tense or anxious. Eating too fast also means that food reaches the gut in bigger lumps, which means it remains there for longer, ferments and produces gas. Some people also suffer from bloating when they eat certain cereals, fruit or vegetables. It's thought that for some people digesting the fibre and sugars in these foods produces wind and bloating.

Not drinking enough fluids can also cause bloating, because dehydration causes an imbalance in electrolytes (body salts) which can slow down digestion.

Bad breath
This can be a sign of digestive problems. Poorly digested food can putrefy in the intestines, producing noxious gases that travel back up to your mouth causing bad breath.

Constipation

Constipation is where having a bowel movement is more difficult, or happens less often than usual. Normal bowel habits vary from one person to another. Some people go to the toilet more than once a day while others may only go once every three or four days. Your poo may be hard or lumpy and you may feel as though you haven't fully emptied your bowel. Other symptoms can include tummy ache and cramps, bloating, nausea and not feeling hungry.

Constipation can be due to diet and lifestyle factors, like not eating enough fibre or drinking enough fluids, lack of exercise, a hectic schedule where you don't make time to go to the toilet, pregnancy, or certain medications and medical conditions. Stress, depression and anxiety can also affect bowel habits.

Going to the loo – what's normal?
People often think they should have a bowel movement every day, but what is 'normal' can vary from one person to another. Most people will have a bowel movement between three times a day and three times a week. If you find yourself going to the loo less often than usual you may be constipated. Another sign is if the stools are hard and pellet-like, rather than soft and well formed.

When to seek medical help
Everyone has gut problems from time to time. But if you have any of the symptoms below for more than a few days for no obvious reason, you're advised to seek medical advice – please don't self-diagnose!

- Tummy pain before or after meals
- Feeling full or bloated
- Nausea or vomiting
- Heartburn or regurgitation
- Pain or problems swallowing
- Appetite loss
- Unexplained weight loss
- Indigestion, especially if for the first time or in mid or later life
- Diarrhoea, constipation or any persistent change in bowel habits
- Black, tarry stools
- Blood or blood and mucus in your poo

- Pain when you have a poo
- A swelling or lump in your stomach or back passage
- Feeling tired, lethargic, feverish or generally unwell

If you see your doctor when you have any of these symptoms, it's likely they'll want to investigate the cause by doing a few tests.

Blood sample

They may take a blood sample to check for anaemia, inflammation in the body or coeliac disease. Coeliac disease is a condition where nutrients and fluids are not absorbed because the intestinal wall is damaged by the immune system reacting to the proteins in cereals like wheat, rye and barley. See **Chapter 3** for more information.

Colonoscopy

They may take a stool sample to see if there's any blood in it. More advanced tests, such as a colonoscopy – where a special telescopic camera is used to see inside the bowel to check for inflammation or early signs of bowel cancer – are usually only carried out if you are over 45 or have symptoms like blood in your poo, unexplained weight loss or a swelling in the stomach or back passage, or if you have a family history of bowel or ovarian cancer. If there's inflammation it may be a sign of inflammatory bowel disease (IBD), a term mainly used to describe two long-term health issues – ulcerative colitis and Crohn's disease. Both conditions can cause an inflamed colon and other symptoms like bloody diarrhoea, tummy pain, fatigue and unexplained weight loss.

Ulcerative colitis

Ulcerative colitis only affects the rectum (back passage) and colon (large intestine). It's thought to be an autoimmune condition. This is where the immune system mistakenly identifies healthy tissue as a foreign invader and attacks it. When the immune system fights off an infection it releases white blood cells into the bloodstream to destroy the foreign invader. This causes swelling and redness, known as inflammation. In ulcerative colitis the immune system mistakenly identifies friendly gut bacteria in the large intestine as a harmful infection and attacks them, causing inflammation in the colon and rectum. Some experts think the condition is caused by an imbalance between the good and bad bacteria in the gut.

Crohn's disease

Crohn's disease is also an autoimmune disorder where the gut lining is inflamed. It can affect any part of the gut but most commonly affects the small or large intestine. As in ulcerative colitis, in Crohn's the immune system mistakes beneficial bacteria as harmful and attacks them.

Rectal prolapse

Abdominal pain and constipation that don't improve with changes in the diet or laxatives could mean you have a rectal prolapse. This is common in women, especially after childbirth when the pelvic muscles are weakened and don't support the rectum. The rectum then collapses, preventing the sufferer from passing a stool. This condition can be hard to pick up, because the rectum usually collapses internally.

Other tests

Your GP may also carry out tests to exclude other causes of tummy pain or discomfort such as diverticular disease, chronic pancreatitis, gallstones, peptic ulcer disease, cholecystitis (inflammation of the gall bladder) and gastro-oesophageal reflux disease (symptoms caused by stomach acid travelling up to the throat).

IBS

If the results of these tests exclude all of the above potentially serious conditions, it's likely your GP will diagnose irritable bowel syndrome (IBS).

This is the name given to a range of symptoms caused by a disturbance of the large intestine. These include tummy pain, bloating, diarrhoea and constipation. It affects up to one in three of the UK population at some point in their lives, but it usually first develops during the teens and early adulthood. It's often a chronic condition, though the symptoms can change or disappear, then return later on.

The ABC of IBS

The National Institute for Clinical Excellence (NICE) recommends that anyone reporting any of these symptoms for at least six weeks should be assessed for IBS:

- **A**bdominal pain and discomfort
- **B**loating
- **C**hange in bowel habits (diarrhoea or constipation)

While IBS isn't life-threatening, it can severely disrupt daily life. Having to dash to the loo often while at work, travelling or socialising is inconvenient and embarrassing. The symptoms can vary from mild to severe. Some people only suffer occasionally – perhaps only when they eat a particular food – while others experience symptoms so severe they regularly have to take time off work and even an everyday shopping trip can be a nightmare.

How common is IBS?

Around 20 per cent of people are thought to suffer from IBS at any one time. But only around one in ten people will see their GP about IBS-type symptoms, as most people find talking about their bowel problems too embarrassing, or think their symptoms will eventually go away on their own. Up to three times as many women have IBS symptoms as men. Around 45 per cent of women with IBS report worsening symptoms just before and during their monthly period. This could be because there are receptors for female hormones in the gut lining, suggesting they have a role in regulating gut function. It's also more common in the Western world, which suggests that IBS, like many health problems of the twenty-first century, is linked to a stressful lifestyle, as well as an over-reliance on fatty, sugary, refined foods and a lack of exercise.

How to beat IBS

So while IBS can have a negative impact on your life, it's not a serious condition. It can largely be managed by following the advice in this book, which will help you achieve a healthy gut through eating the right foods, managing stress, following good sleep habits and taking regular exercise.

Insoluble fibre (roughage) and an overgrowth of unhealthy bacteria such as *E. coli* and *Clostridia* in the gut often contribute to IBS symptoms. These 'bad' bacteria give off excessive amounts of gases and toxic waste products when they ferment food residues in the bowel, causing wind, bloating, pain and diarrhoea. This is known as malfermentation.

If you are diagnosed with IBS you should find especially helpful the advice on which type of fibre to eat in **Chapter 2** and how to boost the good bacteria in your gut in **Chapter 7**.

Other signs of an unhealthy gut

Other signs of an unhealthy gut include weight gain, type 2 diabetes, skin conditions, mental health problems and other issues linked to inflammation, such as arthritis and heart disease.

How your gut flora can make you fat

A healthy diet with plenty of fruit and vegetables and fermented foods like cheese, yogurt and sauerkraut introduces and promotes good gut bacteria like *Akkermansia*, *Bacteroidetes* and *Lactobacillus*, which are linked with health and well-being. See **Chapter 7** to learn more about these beneficial bugs.

On the other hand, eating a lot of sugary and processed foods is linked with less beneficial bacteria – such as *Firmicutes* – that can have a negative impact on your health. A 2013 Spanish study found that *Firmicutes* (and other bacteria linked to weight gain) lowered levels of leptin, a hormone that tells us when we're full, and raised levels of the hunger hormone ghrelin, which led to overeating. People who don't get enough sleep also tend to have more *Firmicutes*. See **Chapter 8** to find out more.

Firmicutes are very good at breaking down the food we eat, which means we absorb more calories that we then store as fat. This may have been a good thing when food was in short supply, as it meant we could survive on less, but it's not helpful nowadays when food is plentiful.

Also, the glucose (sugar) from these foods is easily absorbed, so your blood sugar surges rapidly only to fall again just as quickly. This means you feel hungry again soon afterwards and crave more easily digested starchy and sugary foods, creating a vicious cycle that leads to weight gain – especially around the middle.

Other bacteria – such as *Lactobacilli* and *Bifidobacteria* – are less efficient at extracting energy from food, which means more calories are excreted, rather than stored as fat. Research suggests that one particular strain of *Lactobacillus* – *Lactobacillus gasseri*, found in fermented foods – can help with weight loss, especially with fat around the middle which is linked with a high risk of type 2 diabetes. But other strains have also been shown to help. So a wholesome diet that includes fermented foods is a good weapon against weight gain and associated health problems.

Type 2 diabetes and gut health

Eating a lot of refined carbohydrates, like white pasta, bread and rice, cakes and biscuits and sugary foods, not only affects the healthy balance of gut bacteria, but also raises the risk of type 2 diabetes.

In type 2 diabetes either the pancreas can't produce enough insulin or the body's cells become resistant (don't react) to it.

The diagram on page 25 helps explain how a poor diet raises the risk of weight gain, insulin resistance and, eventually, type 2 diabetes.

How refined and sugary foods are linked to type 2 diabetes

When you eat a lot of white bread, white rice, pasta, crisps, cakes, biscuits and sweets

Unhealthy bacteria, e.g. firmicutes, flourish

Blood sugar spikes rapidly

Firmicutes digest food more efficiently, so more calories absorbed

Pancreas releases insulin which enables cells to use sugar for energy

More calories likely to be stored as fat – especially around middle

Frequent blood sugar spikes cause pancreas to pump out more and more insulin

Belly fat releases inflammatory chemicals called cytokines, linked with insulin resistance

Cells respond less to insulin = insulin resistance and more energy stored as fat

Pancreas has to make more and more insulin, until it can't keep up

Excess sugar (glucose) builds up in bloodstream

Leading to pre-diabetes and type 2 diabetes

Inside out: how your gut bacteria can affect your skin

Unhealthy skin can also be an outward sign of an unhealthy gut. Growing evidence suggests that skin conditions like acne, eczema and rosacea are signs that the balance between healthy and unhealthy gut bacteria is out of kilter. As well as a diet of largely refined, processed, sugary foods and little fibre and nutrients, stress can play a part.

A poor diet of processed and sugary foods combined with stress can allow unhealthy bacteria to thrive, causing damage to the gut lining. This results in what's known as 'leaky gut syndrome', which can manifest as a flare up of acne, eczema or psoriasis.

What is leaky gut syndrome?

This is where the gut lining becomes inflamed and porous, which allows undigested food particles, bacteria, toxins and germs to leak through into the bloodstream. Here they trigger the immune response which causes inflammation throughout the body. Remember – inflammation is where the immune system releases chemicals to fend off foreign invaders, such as infections, causing redness, heat, swelling and pain. As well as skin problems, chronic inflammation is linked to food allergies, asthma, hay fever, migraine and autoimmune conditions like rheumatoid arthritis. Chronic inflammation of the gut can cause IBS, Crohn's and ulcerative colitis. More serious health problems now being linked with chronic inflammation in the body include depression, type 2 diabetes, heart disease and Alzheimer's.

A lack of good gut bacteria also means we're less likely to break down our food properly and obtain the nutrients we need for healthy skin, such as fatty acids and B vitamins.

How a grumpy gut can make you grumpy

Given the extent to which our gut bacteria influence our physical health, it's not surprising there's growing evidence that they affect our mind too. As mentioned earlier, microbiota in our gut produce various hormones. Some of these hormones – serotonin, dopamine, and gamma-aminobutyric acid (GABA) – regulate our mood. Around half of our dopamine and most of our serotonin are made in the gut, so a lack of beneficial microbes will mean we don't produce enough of these mood-boosting hormones.

Gut bacteria also make other chemicals that affect the brain, including a fatty acid called butyrate, which has been shown to ease anxiety and depression. It's thought these chemicals travel to the brain via the enteric system or 'second brain'. We'll talk more about butyrate later on.

The types of gut bacteria that are good for mental health are thought to include strains of *Lactobacillus, Bifidobacterium, Enterococcus* and certain strains of *Streptococcus*. Some studies have shown that eating foods that boost these types of bacteria can reduce stress and anxiety. For more information on which foods to eat to boost your good gut microbes, see **Chapter 7**.

Do you really need that antibiotic?

Antibiotics can save lives. But it's important to only take them when you really need to, as they not only kill off the bacteria behind an infection, but the good bacteria in your gut as well. Remember, antibiotics only work on bacterial infections, not viral ones like colds and flu. After a course of antibiotics it's a good idea to reboot your microbiome (or biome for short) with probiotics, either by eating fermented foods (see **Chapter 7**) or by taking a good-quality probiotic supplement (see **Resources**). Non-steroidal anti-inflammatory drugs (NSAIDs) like ibuprofen and aspirin can also harm your gut health. If taken regularly, they can damage the gut lining because they block chemicals that heal the gut as well as those that cause pain. Taking them with food can help protect the gut.

In a nutshell: signs and causes of an unhealthy gut

- An unhealthy lifestyle can have a negative impact on your gut health.

- Poor gut health can affect both your physical and mental well-being.

- Signs of an unhealthy gut include digestive problems, weight gain, type 2 diabetes, skin problems and low mood.

- See your GP about persistent digestive symptoms, as they could signal more serious conditions like coeliac disease or Crohn's disease.

PART 2

FOOD AND THE GUT

CHAPTER 2
FILL UP ON FIBRE

Your body can't digest fibre but your gut bacteria can, so eating plenty of fibre-rich foods – such as fruit, vegetables, pulses (e.g. baked beans, kidney beans, chickpeas) and wholegrains – will help your good gut bacteria to flourish. Some fruits and vegetables contain prebiotic fibre which acts like a fertiliser for gut bacteria. You'll find more information about prebiotics in **Chapter 7**. A diet high in fibre offers other gut health benefits, including reducing the risk of constipation, piles, diverticular disease and bowel cancer. The NHS recommends that we have 30 g of fibre daily but most people only eat about 18 g.

Diverticular disease
Diverticular disease occurs when little bulges develop in the large intestine and become inflamed. The condition is linked with not eating enough fibre, leading to constipation. Pushing small, hard lumps of poo through your colon can put extra pressure on the gut lining, causing weak areas where the gut lining bulges through to form small pouches called diverticula. Sometimes bacteria can get

trapped inside one of the pouches causing a more severe condition called diverticulitis. Eating plenty of fibre can both prevent diverticular disease and improve symptoms.

The two types of fibre

There are two types of fibre – soluble and insoluble (roughage). Most plant foods contain a mixture of the two. Soluble fibre is mainly found in plant cells and insoluble fibre is found in the plant cell walls. Soluble fibre dissolves to form a gel when it mixes with liquid in the gut. Insoluble fibre doesn't dissolve in liquid so it's especially good for preventing constipation. High-fibre foods are classified according to whether they contain more soluble or insoluble fibre.

Which foods contain soluble fibre?

- Wholegrains such as oats, barley and rye
- Starchy vegetables like potatoes, sweet potatoes, parsnips and carrots
- Pulses like beans, peas and lentils
- Fruits, including apples, pears, bananas and strawberries

Which foods contain insoluble fibre?

- Wholegrain cereals, such as wholemeal bread, wholewheat and bran cereals, and brown rice and pastas
- The skins of fruit and vegetables
- Nuts and seeds

Both types of fibre provide bulk, which stimulates the bowel to push food through the gut, helping to prevent constipation. Fibre also absorbs water from the gut, which makes the stools bigger and softer and therefore easier to pass. Fibre also helps protect your gut from the harmful effects of eating red meat (see **Chapter 6**). As fibre 'feeds' bacteria, it increases their numbers, which means that more are passed out in your poo. This is another reason why fibre makes your poo bulkier. For good gut health, you need to include both types of fibre in your diet. But if you suffer from IBS-D – which means your IBS symptoms include diarrhoea – you may find insoluble fibre makes it worse.

Fibre and IBS

If you have IBS-D, eating less insoluble fibre and more soluble fibre may help ease your symptoms. Soluble fibre is less likely to irritate the gut lining, or cause wind and bloating, because it's broken down quickly. Replace wholemeal bread, wholewheat cereals and wholegrain rice with foods high in soluble fibre, such as oat bread, porridge, oatcakes, barley and pulses.

Fibre providers

To give you an idea of what to eat to get your 30 g of fibre a day, below are examples of the foods and portion sizes that provide approximately 5 g fibre. In all cases, wholegrain versions of cereals, pastas and rice provide the most fibre. The skins of fruit and vegetables are especially high in insoluble fibre, so eat them whenever you can. Where there is a refined (white) version, I've compared the amount you'd need to eat to get the same amount of fibre.

- 2 Weetabix (or four 30 g servings of cornflakes)
- 2 slices wholemeal bread (or six slices white bread)
- 3 rye crispbreads
- 150 g (uncooked weight) brown rice (or 1.2 kg white rice)
- 80 g (uncooked weight) wholewheat pasta (or around 240 g white pasta)
- 1 medium (180 g) baked potato including the skin (or 450 g mashed potato)
- ⅓ 415 g tin of baked beans
- ½ cup of cooked sweetcorn
- 2 medium oranges, pears, apples or bananas
- 45 g (3 tbsp) frozen peas

In a nutshell: why you should fill up on fibre
- Both soluble and insoluble fibre help your gut bacteria to flourish.
- Fibre also helps prevent digestive problems and bowel cancer.
- The NHS recommends having 30 g a day, but most people only eat about 18 g.

CHAPTER 3

GET TO GRIPS
WITH GLUTEN

Gluten is a type of protein in wheat, barley and rye. It's found in foods that contain these grains, such as bread, breakfast cereals, biscuits, cakes, pasta, ready meals and sauces. It can cause digestive problems for some people in the form of coeliac disease and gluten sensitivity.

Coeliac disease

Coeliac disease is a serious condition that affects around 1 in 100 people. While you can develop it in childhood, the most common age of diagnosis is between 40 and 60. It isn't caused by a gluten allergy or intolerance. It's a lifelong condition – once you're diagnosed you'll always have to avoid gluten.

In coeliac disease the body's immune system mistakes gluten as a threat and attacks it. This damages the villi – small finger-like projections that increase the surface area and help nutrient uptake from the small intestine. This prevents the body from absorbing nutrients properly. When sufferers eat foods containing gluten, they can suffer from:

Digestive symptoms
- Diarrhoea (foul smelling)
- Tummy pain
- Bloating
- Wind
- Indigestion
- Constipation

Other symptoms
- Fatigue (from not getting enough nutrients)
- Unexplained weight loss
- An itchy rash
- Fertility problems
- Nerve damage
- Coordination, balance and speech problems

Going gut-friendly gluten-free

Following a gut-friendly gluten-free diet might seem daunting at first but the tips below should make it easier.

1. **Base your diet on naturally gluten-free, gut-friendly foods**, such as fresh fruit and vegetables, fish, poultry, meat, cheese and eggs. Choose naturally gluten-free grains, cereals and foods such as quinoa, rice noodles, polenta, buckwheat, millet, corn and tapioca.

2. **Check food labels** – according to UK law if a cereal that contains gluten has been used in a product it must be listed in the ingredients. While most natural and Greek yogurts are gluten-free, some flavoured varieties may contain gluten. Be especially vigilant with sauces, gravies and condiments, as many contain wheat flour.

3. **Use gluten-free alternatives** – gluten-free pasta, bread, crackers and cereals are widely available in supermarkets, so you needn't deprive yourself of these foods. Some gluten-free staples are available on prescription from the NHS. Bear in mind though that these foods tend to contain more sugar and other additives to make them taste better.

4. **Minimise the risk of cross-contamination** – wipe down kitchen surfaces before preparing your meals and use your own separate butter, cheese, jams and spreads to reduce the risk of ingesting crumbs from foods containing gluten that other members of the household eat.

5. **Adapt your favourite recipes** – there's no need to stop cooking your favourite dishes or avoid trying new gut-friendly ones (such as the ones in this book!). Simply swap gluten-containing ingredients for gluten-free versions.

6. **Choose gluten-free alcoholic drinks**, such as cider, wine and spirits, but avoid beers, lagers, stouts and ales, as these all contain gluten. Spirits made from grains – such as whiskey, which is made from barley – are gluten-free because the gluten proteins are removed during distillation.

Non-coeliac gluten sensitivity (NCGS)

This is where people experience the same digestive problems as people with coeliac disease, but there's no damage to the gut. It's hard to diagnose, as there are no tests.

Coeliac UK recommends that if you have symptoms after eating wheat, barley or rye, you shouldn't try a gluten-free diet straightaway, but should see your GP so that you can be tested for coeliac disease first. It's important you keep eating gluten to make sure the test is accurate. If your test results rule out coeliac disease you could speak to your GP about NCGS and the possibility of cutting out gluten to see if your symptoms improve. Coeliac UK (see **Resources**) offers advice and support on following a gluten-free diet.

A lot of people seem to be opting for gluten-free alternatives to everyday bread and cakes etc. under the illusion that they are somehow healthier. However, as we've already mentioned, many of these have extra additives to make them more palatable, so unless you really do have a problem digesting gluten, they are best avoided.

NCGS - new findings

New research suggests that gluten may not be the problem for some people diagnosed with NCGS. Some people's symptoms may be caused by another type of protein found in wheat, barley and rye called amylase-trypsin inhibitors (ATIs). Although ATIs make up only 4 per cent of wheat proteins, they've been linked to strong immune reactions that can spread from the intestines to other parts of the body. It's also thought ATIs may exacerbate symptoms of rheumatoid arthritis, MS, asthma, lupus and inflammatory bowel disease (IBD). Because of this new research NCGS may be renamed if gluten is shown not to be the main trigger after all.

In a nutshell: get to grips with gluten

- Gluten is a type of protein found in wheat, barley and rye.
- In coeliac disease the immune system wrongly attacks gluten, damaging the small intestine.
- You can still enjoy your favourite foods and eat a gut-friendly diet while avoiding gluten.
- Non-coeliac gluten sensitivity (NCGS) also causes symptoms, but doesn't harm the gut.

CHAPTER 4

SUGAR – NOT SO SWEET

Eating too much sugar has recently been blamed for a litany of health issues, including weight problems, type 2 diabetes, heart disease and stroke (cardiovascular disease), as well as tooth decay, gum disease and ageing skin. Also, people who eat a lot of sugar tend to have a low intake of important nutrients, such as vitamins A and C, folic acid, vitamin B12, calcium, phosphorous, magnesium and iron. This is probably because filling up on sugary foods leaves less appetite or room for more nutritious foods.

Eating a lot of sugar is also bad for the biome. 'Bad' gut bacteria love refined sugars and if you eat too many they can multiply, pushing out the 'good' bacteria you need for a healthy gut.

This chapter explains what sugar is, why we crave it and how to curb our cravings and eat less to benefit our biome and overall health.

Some people also have problems digesting fructose, while others have trouble breaking down lactose, so we'll also look at these issues.

The low-down on sugar

There are several different types of sugar, including lactose, glucose and fructose. Lactose is the sugar found in milk. Glucose is found naturally in fruit and vegetables, pulses and grains. Fructose is found naturally in fruit and honey, and to a lesser degree in vegetables. Sucrose is the man-made, refined sugar commonly added to foods and drinks. It's extracted from sugar cane and sugar beet and contains both glucose and fructose.

Do we need sugar in our diets?

While our brain and body need a steady supply of glucose to function properly, we can get all of our daily glucose needs from eating a balanced diet containing fruit, vegetables, pulses and wholegrains. Also, we turn some of the protein and fat we eat into glucose: all natural foods provide your body with glucose, so you don't need to eat extra sugar!

Why we crave sugar

This need for glucose helps explain why we crave sugar. Add to that the fact that refined sugar gives you a quick burst of energy. This is because sucrose is easily converted into glucose, which is quickly absorbed into the bloodstream. When the blood sugar rises too high, too rapidly, the body reacts by producing insulin, which lowers it by directing glucose to the body's cells. Our blood sugar then plummets and we crave another sugar 'hit'.

Sugar is also addictive, because when we eat it our brain releases dopamine, a 'feel good' hormone. If we eat sugar every day our brains stop producing as much dopamine in response, so we have to eat more and more to get the same pleasurable feelings. So the more sugar you eat, the more you crave.

Curb sugar cravings

Eating a diet rich in fruit and vegetables, wholegrains, proteins and healthy fats, rather than refined foods, is the best way to curb sugar cravings. Fruit and vegetables supply sugars in their natural form, along with other nutrients, whereas sucrose has no nutritional value. It takes the body longer to break down the sugars (fructose and glucose) in fruit, vegetables and wholegrains because of the fibre they contain. And, of course, the fibre they contain supplies prebiotics to help your good gut bacteria to thrive.

Proteins and fats slow down the rate at which the body digests sugars. This means that when you eat foods containing them your blood sugar remains steady for longer, avoiding the highs and lows caused by eating refined carbs and sugars. So try to include sources of protein and healthy fats, such as fish, seafood, poultry, eggs, meat, natural yogurt, oats, pulses, nuts and seeds and small amounts of olive or rapeseed oil, butter or avocado, in your meals as often as you can.

Happy gut tip

To help beat sugar cravings try sniffing a bottle of vanilla essence. Many people find it reduces the urge to eat sweet foods. Cinnamon also helps and it steadies the blood sugar. Try it sprinkled over porridge, stewed fruit or a latte.

Sweet enough

NHS Choices recommends we eat no more than 30 g of added sugars a day, which is roughly the equivalent of six teaspoons. This might sound like quite a lot until you realise that a can of fizzy cola can have 35 g of sugar in it, or that a small 45 g milk chocolate bar can contain up to 25 g. But it's not just sweet foods and drinks that have added sugar – so do savoury items like soups, baked beans, bread, crisps, cooking sauces, salad creams and ready-made meals.

Eat less sugar

The best way to eat less sugar is to avoid processed foods or at least keep them down to a minimum. Realistically, we'll all eat these foods from time to time, but you can still keep your sugar intake in check if you look at the sugar content and opt for those products that contain less sugar.

How to check food labels

Unfortunately this isn't as easy as it sounds because food manufacturers are not legally obliged to specify what type of sugar is in their product. So all they give is a figure under the heading 'Carbohydrate (of which sugars)'. This means when a label says 'sugars' it's referring to all of the different types of sugar in the product, both naturally occurring (from fruit, vegetables and milk) and added. That's why it's a good idea to check the ingredients list for added sugars. We will look at this in more detail shortly.

How can I tell if a food is high or low in sugar?

According to the Food Standards Agency, if a food product contains less than 5 g of sugar per 100 g it is low in sugar. If a product contains more than 22.5 g of sugar per 100 g it is high in sugar.

Some foods also have labels on the front to give a quick guide to their nutritional content, so you can compare different products at a glance. Some are also colour-coded, to make it even easier to determine whether a food is high in sugar, with red meaning high, amber meaning medium and green meaning low. But be aware that a manufacturer's portion may be different to the amount you actually eat. For example, the label on a can of fizzy pop will tell you how much sugar there is in 100 ml, but the can will contain 330 ml, so you will have to multiply the amount given by 3.3 to find out the total amount of sugar in it.

Sugar by any other name

When you check labels for added sugar, be aware of the other guises it comes under. If you spot any of these names you will know sugars have been added. The main ingredients always come first, so if any of these are near the top of the list, avoid the product.

- Agave
- Agave nectar
- Barley malt syrup
- Beet sugar
- Blackstrap molasses
- Blossom nectar sugar
- Brown rice syrup
- Brown sugar
- Cane sugar
- Caramel
- Carob syrup
- Coconut nectar
- Coconut sugar
- Coconut syrup
- Corn syrup
- Dark muscovado sugar
- Date sugar
- Date syrup
- Dextrin
- Dextrose

- Fructose
- Glucose
- Glucose syrup
- Golden caster sugar
- Golden syrup
- Grape sugar
- High-fructose corn syrup
- Honey
- Hydrolysed starch
- Icing sugar
- Invert sugar
- Invert syrup
- Malt extract
- Malt sugar
- Malt syrup
- Maltose
- Maple syrup
- Molasses
- Organic sugar
- Palm sugar
- Raw sugar
- Saccharose
- Sorghum syrup
- Sucrose
- Sugar beet syrup
- Syrup
- Treacle
- Turbinado sugar

Aka sugar

The word 'syrup' or 'sweetener' or a word ending in '-ose' is just another name for sugar.

Watch out for more than one sugar

Food manufacturers know we check to see if sugar is listed at the top of the ingredients list, so they avoid having to put sugar there by using various forms and listing each one separately. As the sugar content is spread across a few different types of sugar, they are used in smaller amounts and can legitimately be listed further down the ingredients list.

Dairy foods differ

Don't be alarmed if you look at the food label for whole milk (cow, goat or sheep) and see it contains 4.7 g (one teaspoon) of sugar per 100 ml. Remember the sugar in milk is naturally occurring lactose, which is broken down into glucose and galactose. So milk is sucrose-free. Also, lactose is good for most people's guts because it feeds beneficial bacteria like *Lactobacilli* and *Bifidobacteria*. It's only a problem for people with lactose intolerance.

So if you're working out how much sugar is in a milk drink, you can ignore the first 4.7 g of sugar per 100 ml and assume that any figure over 4.7 g is added sugar. For example, if your child's favourite chocolate milk drink has 13 g of sugar per 100 ml in it, you'll know there is 8.3 g of added sugar per 100 ml (13 g – 4.7 g of lactose = 8.3 g). This is equal to around two teaspoons of added sugar.

Other dairy products, such as cheese, cream, butter and yogurt, contain differing amounts of lactose, depending on how they are made. For example, natural yogurt contains on average around 3.5 g of lactose per 100 g. So if the food label on a 120 g pot of fruit yogurt states it contains 12 g of sugars that means it has around 4.2 g of lactose and 7.8 g of added sugar.

Happy gut tip

Yogurt is a fermented food so bacteria break down the lactose, making it easier to digest, which means that some people with lactose intolerance can eat yogurt without suffering any ill effects.

Sweet nothings

Below are some simple ways to cut back on sugar. You don't need to try them all at once. Just introduce one step at a time until eating less sugar becomes second nature.

- Gradually reduce the amount of sugar you add to tea and other drinks until you can do without.

- Avoid 'designer' coffees from coffee shops, as they can contain a lot of sugar. For example, a Starbucks large white chocolate mocha contains up to 76 g of sugar!

- Use cinnamon, ginger, nutmeg, vanilla, cloves, cardamoms or star anise to sweeten desserts, instead of sugar.

- Satisfy your sweet tooth with sweet-tasting vegetables like beetroot, butternut squash, sweet potato, podded peas, sweetcorn, red peppers, cherry tomatoes, pumpkins, carrots and parsnips.

- Replace sugar-coated breakfast cereals with wholegrain cereals like Weetabix or porridge.

- Freeze a banana on a stick for a sweet but healthy alternative to ice cream.

- Choose tinned fruits in natural juice rather than syrup.

- Instead of sweet or stodgy puddings, choose baked apples or summer pudding.

- Replace high-sugar flavoured yogurts with natural yogurt and fresh fruit or canned fruit in fruit juice.

- Use reduced-sugar jams.

- Cut the amount of sugar you use when baking by up to half.

- Avoid cereal bars – despite containing 'healthy' ingredients like honey, they tend to be high in sugar.

- If you can't do without fizzy drinks, try diluting small amounts of unsweetened fruit juice with sparkling water.

- Swap sugary squash or cordial for the no-added-sugar kind.

Are sweeteners better for my gut?

Unfortunately, like sugar, artificial sweeteners such as aspartame, mannitol, sorbitol, stevia, sucralose and xylitol can lead to an overgrowth of bad bacteria that cause inflammation and weight problems, so it's best to avoid them.

Home-made tomato pasta sauce (serves 2)

Replace ready-made pasta sauce (containing added sugar) with a home-made low-sugar version. Fry a finely diced medium white onion in olive oil for 5 minutes. Add 2 cloves of grated garlic and a bunch of fresh basil and fry until they start to brown. Stir in one 350 g jar of tomato passata and one tablespoon of red wine vinegar. Simmer for around 15 minutes, stirring occasionally. Serve with 200 g of cooked wholewheat pasta and some grated parmesan.

Fructose intolerance

Fructose intolerance is not really an intolerance – it's more an inability to absorb fructose. Some people can't completely absorb it in their small intestine, so undigested fructose is carried to the large intestine where gut bacteria devour it. As they do so, the bacteria give off gases which cause wind, bloating, tummy cramps and diarrhoea – classic IBS symptoms.

Fructose intolerance often only happens when sufferers eat too much fructose. The easiest way to overdose on fructose is to eat lots of sugary and processed foods which contain unnaturally high amounts of fructose, compared to say an apple or an orange.

So if you think you have a problem with fructose it's worth cutting back on processed foods to see if that helps.

If you still have symptoms, you may need to avoid high-fructose fruits like apples, pears and grapes and opt for fruits like rhubarb, pineapples, strawberries, blackberries, lemons, limes, avocados and bananas.

Happy gut tip

Try eating stewed or baked apples or poached pears, as these fruits are often easier to digest when cooked.

Lactose intolerance

Lactose is the sugar found in milk. Some people have problems digesting it because they don't make the enzyme lactase to break it down. As a result they suffer from symptoms like diarrhoea, constipation and cramping when they consume milk and milk products. If they eat fermented dairy products – for example, yogurt, cheese and buttermilk – they might not have these symptoms because the bacteria in those foods break down the lactose.

In a nutshell: why sugar is not so sweet

- Sugar added to food and drink is made from glucose and fructose and is called sucrose.

- Too much sugar upsets the healthy balance of gut bacteria.

- Excess sugar is also linked to weight gain, type 2 diabetes, cardiovascular disease, dental problems and poor nutrition.

- When you check labels for sugar content, remember food manufacturers call it many different names.

CHAPTER 5

HEAL YOUR GUT WITH HEALTHY FATS

Fats had a bad press until recently. For years we were told that fats – especially saturated fats – made us fat, caused heart disease and needed to be avoided. Now we know that small amounts of healthy fats are vital for good health and it is refined carbohydrates and sugar that we need to cut back on.

Your brain is approximately 60 per cent fat, so you need it for your brain to function properly. The body also uses fats to make cell membranes and hormones. And you need fats to help you absorb fat-soluble vitamins such as A, D, E and K and keep your hair, skin and nails healthy.

Eating healthy fats can also boost high-density lipoprotein (HDL) cholesterol, which can lower your risk of heart disease. They help keep you lean by making you feel fuller and less likely to crave sugary, starchy foods. They are also good for your gut – helping to soothe and heal the mucous membranes and boost beneficial bugs. There are two main types of fats – saturated and unsaturated.

Saturated fats

Saturated fats are mainly found in animal products such as red meat, butter, whole milk, yogurt and cheese. Experts now believe saturated fats are good for you in small amounts. Recent research found that people who eat full-fat dairy foods generally have better heart health and less risk of type 2 diabetes.

Healthy sources of saturated fats include eggs, whole milk, butter, full-fat natural yogurt and cheeses, organic poultry and meats, coconut, coconut oil and avocado. Butter and cheese are also sources of butyrate, a fat that keeps the gut lining healthy.

Unsaturated fats

There are two types of unsaturated fat – polyunsaturated essential fatty acids (omegas 3 and 6) and monounsaturated fat (omega 9).

These are known as essential fatty acids because they can't be made by the body, so you need to get them from your diet.

Omega 3 fats

Omega 3 fats help to soothe and repair the gut lining and boost beneficial bacteria. Most of us don't eat enough omega 3 fats, so make sure you include these foods in your diet:

- Oily fish, such as pilchards, sardines, salmon and mackerel
- Nuts, especially walnuts, Brazil nuts and almonds
- Seeds, especially chia, sesame and flax
- Oils, including soya bean oil, sunflower oil, canola oil and rapeseed oil
- Egg yolks

Omega 6 fats

Omega 6s are also anti-inflammatory and can help ease the symptoms of IBS. Most people get plenty of these in their diet. They are found in:

- Sunflower and corn oils
- Olives
- Nuts such as hazelnuts, cashews and pistachios
- Seeds such as flaxseeds (linseeds), sunflower and pumpkin
- Some vegetables and grains

Monounsaturated (omega 9) fats

Monounsaturated or omega 9 fats lower bad, low-density lipoprotein (LDL) cholesterol and increase good, HDL cholesterol and calm inflammation in the body. Good sources of monounsaturated fats are:

- Olives and olive oil – also rich in polyphenols, which are natural substances that boost good bacteria
- Rapeseed oil
- Peanut oil
- Avocados – also contain phytosterols, which are anti-inflammatory
- Nuts, especially almonds and Brazil nuts
- Seeds, especially sesame

... and fats to avoid

The fats to avoid are the man-made partially hydrogenated fats and trans fats. These are considered the worst types of fat you can eat, as they are strongly linked with fat around the middle and increased risk of heart attack and stroke. They are made by heating and chemically treating liquid vegetable and seed oils to turn them into solid fats. You'll find them in margarines, processed food (biscuits, pies, cakes, ice cream, pastries) and fast food. Avoid products with hydrogenated fat, hydrogenated vegetable oil, partially hydrogenated vegetable fat/oil or trans fatty acids listed in the ingredients. Research also shows that eating a lot of trans fats has a negative effect on the biome.

Happy gut reminder: butyrate and acetic acid
These are the gut-healing fatty acids that gut bacteria produce from resistant starch found in green (unripe) bananas, beans, chilled pasta, chilled rice and chilled potatoes. So include these foods in your diet as well. **Safety note:** Rice should be cooled and chilled quickly and reheated only once within 24 hours, to avoid the risk of food poisoning.

In a nutshell: fats and the gut

- Far from being bad for us, fats are needed by the body, including the gut, for good health.

- Eat oily fish, grains, nuts, seeds, avocados, olive and rapeseed oils for healthy fats that help heal your gut.

- Avoid man-made partially hydrogenated fats and trans fats – they're linked with unhealthy tummy fat.

CHAPTER 6

WHY YOUR GUT NEEDS PROTEIN

This chapter looks at why protein is vital for a healthy gut, including how it helps gut bacteria to flourish and to produce hormones needed for sound sleep and our emotional and physical well-being.

Building blocks of life

Proteins are an important part of a balanced diet. They're needed for cell growth and tissue repair. All proteins are made up of different combinations of 20 compounds known as amino acids. Depending on the amino acids they contain, proteins are used to make enzymes, hormones, muscles, organs and other tissues in the body. So clearly they're vital for a healthy gut and digestion. There are two types of amino acids:

- **Non-essential amino acids** – which your body can make.
- **Essential amino acids** – which your body can't make and must get from food. There are nine essential amino acids.

Protein types

- **Animal proteins** - contain all nine essential amino acids and are found in meat, poultry, fish, eggs and dairy products.

- **Plant proteins** – contain a range of amino acids. Sources of plant protein include pulses (beans, peas, lentils), cereals, grains (such as oats), nuts and seeds, soya and Quorn.

No single plant source has all of the essential amino acids, so if you're vegetarian or vegan you need to eat a mix of these foods. For example, beans on toast, or cereal with milk (dairy or plant-based, depending on your personal preference).

Protein takes longer for the body to break down. So eating some protein with every meal helps you to stay a healthy weight because it keeps you full for longer. It also helps prevent your blood sugar from rising too quickly.

Proteins also have an impact on gut health. Gut flora need nitrogen from proteins to flourish, as well as to digest fibre and produce short-chain fatty acids like butyrate, which keep your gut lining healthy. Also, when you eat protein-rich foods containing the amino acid tryptophan, your gut bacteria turn it into the 'happy hormone' serotonin. Serotonin is converted into the sleep hormone melatonin at night. Tryptophan-rich foods include poultry, eggs, dairy foods, meat, beans, rice, oats, hummus and wholegrains.

Happy gut tip

The average adult needs around 45–56 g of protein each day. This is the amount of protein in a food, not the weight of the food itself. For example, one egg gives you 7 g of protein. A portion of chicken, steak or fish the size of a deck of cards (around 100 g) has around 20 g of protein. So two portions of meat or fish and one egg would meet your daily protein needs.

Protein-rich foods such as meat, eggs and nuts are also good sources of vitamins and iron. But meat has been linked with bowel cancer over the past few years, so can you eat it as part of a gut-friendly diet?

Can meat be gut-friendly?

It seems that when bacteria break down meat they produce chemicals that can harm the gut lining and raise the risk of bowel cancer. The biggest risk is linked to eating a lot of processed meat, rather than having good-quality organic meat once or twice a week. Processed meat is meat that's been preserved by smoking, curing or salting, or by adding preservatives. Processed meats include bacon, beef burgers, ham, pâté, sausages and salami.

Organic lean meat is a nutritious food that gives you high-quality protein which is needed to repair the gut lining. It also supplies gut-soothing omega 3 fats and stress-busting B vitamins, as well as iron and zinc. Cutting meat out altogether could cause anaemia – especially in women.

Evidence suggests that eating plenty of fibre seems to protect against the possible harmful effects of eating red meat. So the message seems to be:

'Eat red meat in moderation, eat plenty of fibre and avoid processed meats as much as possible.' Current guidelines from the Department of Health are to eat no more than 500 g of red meat a week. That's five 100 g servings a week. A 100 g portion is about the size of the palm of your hand and the depth of a deck of cards.

What's classed as red meat?
Red meat includes fresh, minced and frozen beef, lamb, pork and veal, but not poultry or fish.

Is meat hard to digest?

Meat is harder to digest than other foods. It's animal muscle, so you need to chew it more and produce more acid and enzymes to break it down in the gut. It's also high in protein, which again takes longer to digest, but that means it keeps you full for longer so it can help you keep in trim.

Did you know?
Your body naturally prefers cooked foods because they're easier to digest than raw ones. In the case of meat, slow cooking it makes it more tender and easier for your gut to break down.

In a nutshell: your gut and protein

- Your gut needs protein to repair itself and to make enzymes.

- Gut bacteria need protein to grow and make butyrate (a short-chain fatty acid) which boosts gut health.

- Too much red and processed meat is linked with bowel cancer.

- Good-quality meat eaten in moderation and combined with a high-fibre intake can be good for your gut.

PART 3

BALANCE YOUR BIOME

CHAPTER 7
EAT YOUR GUT HAPPY

To eat your gut happy aim for a balanced diet that includes a wide range of fruit, vegetables, wholegrains, pulses (e.g. baked beans, kidney beans and chickpeas) and legumes (e.g. peas and green beans), nuts, seeds and fermented foods such as yogurt and cheese, as well as fish (especially oily), poultry, eggs and a small amount of red meat. We've already discussed the digestive and health problems that sugary and refined, processed foods can cause, so keep these to a minimum. Such a diet will help to boost the range and levels of good bacteria in your gut and keep your gut lining healthy. You shouldn't have to wait long to feel the benefits. According to a 2013 report in *Nature*, if you change your diet – for instance by eating more fibre and less sugar – your gut biome will change within three or four days.

Recent research shows that there is a two-way relationship between our diet and gut bacteria. The food you eat affects the types of bacteria in your gut and they in turn may even influence the food choices you make. It seems they generate cravings for foods they specialise in digesting. So once you start making healthier food choices it should become easier as the healthier bacteria increase.

In this chapter you'll learn about probiotics and which foods are the best sources. You'll also find out about prebiotics and how they help good gut bacteria to flourish.

The low-down on probiotics

Probiotics have become a hot health topic in recent years, with all sorts of claims made about them, but what are they, what do they do and where can you find them?

What are probiotics?

According to the World Health Organization (WHO), probiotics are 'live micro-organisms which, when administered in adequate amounts, confer a health benefit on the host'.

In simpler terms, probiotics are live 'good' bacteria and yeasts that can benefit your health, including your digestion, weight, skin and even your mood. 'Probiotic' literally means 'for life'. Good bacteria are found naturally in fermented foods. Fermented foods are made by using bacteria to change sugars into acid. Fermenting was a commonly used method of preserving food before the introduction of fridges.

Feast on fermented foods

Fermented foods can be made from milk, vegetables, soya, wheat or rye. To reach your intestines, where they can do you good, probiotics have to survive the hydrochloric acid in your stomach and bile in your small intestine. The bacteria in fermented foods are thought to survive stomach acids because they are used to being in an acidic environment.

You can buy fermented foods in the shops but many are pasteurised, to make sure they're safe and to extend their shelf life. Unfortunately, pasteurisation can kill off the beneficial microbes. So if you want to try fermented foods to boost your gut health, look for products that have been made using traditional preparation and processing methods, or make them yourself, to ensure you actually get the healthy bacteria.

Probiotic yogurt drinks such as Yakult and Actimel both contain strains of *Lactobacillus*. Actimel also contains *Streptococcus thermophilus*. However, these drinks can be high in sugar and may contain fructose. The light versions contain sweeteners which, as we saw in **Chapter 1**, can promote 'bad' gut bacteria, so you are probably better off adding naturally probiotic fermented foods to your diet.

Happy gut tip

Probiotic supplements may be useful to repopulate your gut with beneficial bugs after you've taken a course of antibiotics. But some of these can be expensive and not all of them are effective. So, if you can, buy a brand that has been proven to work in clinical trials, such as ProVen and OptiBac (see **Resources**). Some probiotic supplements also have prebiotics such as inulin or fructooligosaccharides (FOS) added to help the bacteria thrive in the gut.

Some of the most studied health benefits of probiotics are:

- Strengthening the immune system to help fend off infection

- Relieving IBS and inflammatory bowel disease (IBD)
- Helping prevent food allergies in children
- Lowering blood cholesterol levels
- Helping prevent tummy bugs
- Improving digestion of lactose in dairy foods

Fermented milk foods

Milk is used to produce fermented products like natural yogurt, kefir (a type of fermented milk) and certain cheeses. They usually contain various strains of *Lactobacilli* and *Bifidobacteria* which seem to work together to improve health, or a strain called *Streptococcus thermophilus*. These probiotics help ease diarrhoea and, as they turn lactose into lactic acid, can help with lactose intolerance. As we saw in **Chapter 1**, some strains of these bacteria also seem to help prevent weight gain.

Note: avoid heating probiotic foods if you can, as it destroys the beneficial bacteria.

Yogurt

Natural yogurt is made by fermenting milk using live bacteria such as *Lactobacilli* and *Bifidobacteria*, which are known as the culture. These bacteria change lactose (the milk sugar) into lactic acid, which thickens the milk and gives it its characteristic tangy flavour.

Full-fat natural yogurt: the most effective probiotic

A 2016 Channel 4 *Food Unwrapped* programme tested a probiotic dark chocolate, unpasteurised sauerkraut, kimchi, a probiotic yogurt drink and full-fat natural yogurt to find out which provided the most bacteria to survive stomach acids, enzymes and bile and reach the intestines. The bacteria found to survive best were from full-fat natural yogurt. The study concluded that this was because the fat protected the bacteria from the acids. Home-made natural yogurt is believed to give you the most probiotics. You can find out how to make your own in **Chapter 11**.

Kefir

Kefir is a cultured, fermented milk drink, which originates from Eastern Europe. It's a natural yogurt drink with a tart, sour taste and a slight fizz from the fermentation process. The length of time it's fermented for affects the taste. Kefir is a good source of calcium and B vitamins and is rich in probiotic bacteria.

The word 'kefir' comes from the old Turkish word *keyif* meaning 'good feeling'. The drink is made by adding kefir 'grains' to a dairy, nut or plant milk. It can be made from cow, ewe, goat or buffalo milk. The grains are small, jelly-like beads that contain up to 50 types of live bacteria – including different strains of *Lactobacillus* (mainly *Lactobacillus kefiri*) – and yeasts which ferment the milk, making kefir one of the most probiotic-rich drinks you can get. The drink is thought to have originated when Caucasian shepherds stored milk in leather bags, where it was fermented by natural bacteria and yeasts.

Kefir is better for the gut than a probiotic drink

According to a 2016 study by the BBC programme *Trust Me, I'm a Doctor*, drinking kefir is one of the best ways to boost your levels of good bacteria. Three groups of ten volunteers each tried a different approach to boosting their beneficial gut bacteria. One group tried a probiotic drink, another ate lots of foods containing the prebiotic inulin and the third group drank kefir. After four weeks those who tried the probiotic drink had a small increase in friendly flora. Those who ate the prebiotics saw a bigger rise in their beneficial bugs. But those who drank the kefir had the biggest increase of helpful microbes. The study concluded that this was because the bacteria in kefir are used to an acidic environment, so they can survive stomach acids to reach the intestines.

You can buy kefir in Polish and larger supermarkets, or you can make your own. See **Chapter 11** to find out how.

Cheese

Cheese is made in a similar way to yogurt. Bacteria are added to sour and thicken the milk, before rennet or lactic acid is added to form curds, which are then matured to form cheese. The bacteria in cheese have been shown to release butyrate, an anti-inflammatory fatty acid that keeps the gut walls healthy. Not all cheeses contain live bacteria, as they can be killed off during the cheese-making process, but the ones listed on page 66 provide decent amounts of beneficial bacteria that survive the journey into the intestines.

Fifteen cheeses that pack the biggest probiotic punch

- Brie
- Cheddar
- Cottage cheese
- Edam
- Emmenthal
- Feta
- Gorgonzola
- Gouda
- Grana Padano
- Gruyère
- Mozzarella
- Parmesan
- Roquefort
- Stilton
- Swiss

Fermented vegetables

Vegetables are naturally covered in *Lactobacillus* bacteria. Fermenting involves pickling them in their own juices or in brine, to allow these bacteria to grow. As the bacteria break down the vegetable sugars, they make lactic acid, which has a vinegary, tangy flavour. The salt and acid stop harmful microbes from growing while enabling the beneficial ones to survive and flourish. When you eat fermented vegetables you benefit not only from the fibre, bacteria and other nutrients, but also, because they've already started breaking down, a gentler digestion process. They also contain prebiotic fibre which helps the bacteria to flourish once they reach your gut. Fermented vegetable foods include sauerkraut, kimchi and olives. Although olives are actually a fruit, I've included them with pickled vegetables because they have a savoury rather than sweet flavour.

Sauerkraut

Sauerkraut is a pickled cabbage, traditionally made in Germany and Poland. It's made by fermenting the cabbage in its own juices and salt. You can buy it in supermarkets but you need to check that it's unpasteurised, as the pasteurisation process kills off the probiotics. It's easy to make at home – find out how in **Chapter 14**.

Kimchi (non-pasteurised)

Kimchi is a traditional Asian pickle that's also made from cabbage with other vegetables and spices. You can buy it in Asian supermarkets and many of the bigger supermarkets. If you want to make your own, you'll find a recipe on page 157.

Olives

Olives are fermented in brine and contain anti-inflammatory olive oil as well as gut-friendly *Lactobacillus*. They're quite salty, but their strong flavour makes you less likely to eat too many.

Happy gut tip

Go for pickles in brine rather than vinegar. Ordinary pickled beetroot, gherkins, red cabbage and onions are preserved in vinegar and are not fermented, so they don't offer the same benefits as those pickled in their own juices or brine.

Fermented soya

Soya is fermented with a range of beneficial yeasts, moulds and bacteria to produce foods like miso, tempeh, nattō, soy or tamari sauce. As with fermented vegetables, the nutrients in fermented soybean products – including protein, omega 3 fats and minerals – are easier to digest and absorb. They also contain plant oestrogens which can help women going through the menopause.

Miso

Miso is a Japanese seasoning made by using a fungus called *Aspergillus oryzae* to ferment soya beans with a grain such as brown or white rice or barley. It has a strong yeasty, savoury flavour and can be added to soups and stews, and rice, fish and meat dishes at the end of cooking when the pan has been removed from the heat, to protect the probiotics it contains. Miso is quite high in salt, but the strong flavour means you only need to use a small amount. For an instant soup, stir a teaspoon into hot water. You can usually buy it in health food stores.

Tempeh

Tempeh is made by inoculating whole cooked soya beans with a type of fungus called *Rhizopus* which grows through the beans and binds them together into a solid cake. It's high in protein and a good source of B vitamins and minerals, making it a good meat substitute. You can eat tempeh with miso or soy sauce or add it to savoury dishes like stir-fries, soups, salads and stews.

Tofu

Tofu is made in a similar way to cheese, only the curds are made from soy milk. Like tempeh, it's high in protein as well as calcium, magnesium and iron. Tofu comes in different textures – extra firm, firm, soft or silken. Firm and extra firm keep their shape when cooked, so they are best for grilling and stir-frying. The soft version works best in soups and casseroles. The silken type is usually used in puddings and dips and can be blended into smoothies for extra protein. Tofu has a neutral taste, which means it absorbs the flavours of whatever you cook it with, so it's very versatile.

Sourdough bread

Ordinary bread is made using store-bought yeast that reacts with gluten to make the dough rise. Sourdough bread is made by adding yeast and bacteria to wheat or rye flour and water, which make lactic acid that ferments the dough. The glucose in sourdough bread takes longer to break down so it keeps you fuller for longer. Also, if you're sensitive to gluten you may find sourdough bread easier to digest than normal bread. If you'd like to try your hand at making your own you'll find a recipe on page 135.

The low-down on prebiotics: what are they?

Prebiotics are a type of plant fibre found in fruit, vegetables, wholegrains and pulses like beans, peas and lentils. Your body can't digest them but they act like a fertiliser, feeding your friendly gut flora, especially *Akkermansia, Bacteroidetes, Bifidobacterium* and *Lactobacillus*.

Because they boost these bacteria, they're linked with these health benefits:

- Fewer tummy bugs
- Relief from Crohn's disease and ulcerative colitis
- Better absorption of calcium and magnesium

- Help you manage your weight
- Lower your risk of bowel cancer

Eat a rainbow

The bigger the variety of colours in the fruit and vegetables you eat, the more diverse your gut biome will be. This is because the different colours in fruit and vegetables signal different plant nutrients (known as phytonutrients). For example, purple fruit and vegetables like blackberries, blueberries, aubergines and red cabbage have anthocyanins that promote the flourishing of friendly flora which help prevent allergies. Green vegetables like broccoli, brussels sprouts, cabbage, kale and spinach contain glucosinolates. When gut bacteria break these down they make substances that help prevent different types of cancer.

Fruit, vegetables and wholegrains contain a range of prebiotics including:

Beta glucan

Beta glucan is a prebiotic fibre found in oats, barley and mushrooms. As well as feeding friendly flora, it lowers 'bad' LDL cholesterol levels in your blood. Because beta glucan is a type of soluble fibre, it forms a gel that cholesterol sticks to. So instead of absorbing it through your gut wall you excrete it.

Inulin

Some fruit and vegetables contain a type of prebiotic known as inulin. Inulins are a type of plant sugar that not only improve digestive health and immunity, but also boost bone strength because they help your body to absorb calcium. They also cut the amount of fat in your bloodstream. They are found in a lot of different plant foods, but Jerusalem artichokes, asparagus, bananas, celery, chickpeas, chicory, cucumber, dandelion greens, garlic, leeks, onions and fresh herbs are especially good sources.

5 a Day

Evidence shows significant health benefits from eating a minimum of five 80 g portions of a variety of fruit and vegetables every day.

The 5 a Day campaign is based on advice from the World Health Organization (WHO), which recommends eating at least 400 g of fruit and vegetables a day to cut the risk of serious health problems. Recent research at Imperial College London found that eating double that amount – ten portions daily – offered the greatest health benefits.

However, it seems that many of us are failing to even meet the lower target. According to a 2017 Diabetes UK survey, two-thirds of UK adults eat only three or less portions of fruit or vegetables a day, while nearly half eat no fruit at least three days a week.

What does 80 g of fruit/vegetables look like?
- Three heaped tablespoons of vegetables
- A handful of fruit – the size of an apple or pear

Easy ways to get your 5 a Day

Find it hard to get your 5 a Day? It's easy once you make it a habit! Here are a few ideas to help you sneak them into your diet:

- Drink fruit juice at breakfast.

- Top your breakfast cereal or porridge with sliced apple or banana, or a few strawberries, raspberries or blueberries.

- Keep a bowl of fruit on show in your kitchen – studies say you're more likely to snack on it.

- Carry a small packet of dried fruit, such as raisins or dried apricots, in your bag.

- Include salad in your lunchtime sandwich.

- Snack on fruit or raw vegetables, such as carrots, celery or peppers. Take some to work.

- Put fruit or raw vegetables on your desk so that you're more likely to eat them.

- Eat raw vegetable sticks with hummus for lunch.

- Have at least two vegetables with your evening meal.

- Add mixed frozen vegetables to chilli con carne or Bolognese sauce near the end of cooking.

- Add fresh fruit to your dessert.

- Make your own soups using your favourite vegetables.

- Add grated carrot, peppers, courgette, celery or beetroot to your spaghetti Bolognese sauce.

- Put lots of chopped vegetables, such as peppers, carrots and onions, into home-made curries.

- Add a handful of berries or chopped fruit to yogurt or hot or cold custard, for a quick and healthy pudding.

- Add halved strawberries or slices of melon, mango or orange to salads.

- If you're too busy to prepare fresh vegetables, have frozen ones instead. They're often more nutritious and still provide prebiotics.

- Frozen fruit or tinned fruit in natural juices are healthy alternatives to fresh fruit.

Resistant starch

Resistant starch is another type of prebiotic. As the name suggests, it's a type of starch that resists digestion in your stomach and small intestine and is virtually still intact when it reaches your large intestine. Here your 'good' gut bacteria digest it. As they do so they release fatty acids such as butyrate, a fatty acid (also found in butter and cheese) that helps to soothe and heal your gut lining, improve the health of your colon (bowel) and cut your risk of colon cancer.

Eating foods containing resistant starch can help you manage your weight too, as your body doesn't digest all of the calories they contain. They're also digested more slowly, so when you eat them you feel full for longer, so you're likely to eat less.

Also, if you suffer from IBS, resistant starch may be a better option than insoluble fibre from wholemeal bread and pasta, as it causes less wind and bloating.

As well as beta glucan, oats and barley contain resistant starch, making them a great source of prebiotics. Uncooked rolled oats – for example, in muesli – are one of the best sources of resistant starch, but cooking them

– for example, when you make porridge – destroys most of it. It can also be found in wheat and in unripe (green) bananas, seeds and legumes, including peas, beans, lentils and peanuts (which belong to the same plant family and are not actually nuts). But there's another way you can boost the amount of resistant starch in your diet.

Why leftovers can be good for your gut!

Resistant starch is also found in potatoes, pasta and rice that have been cooked, chilled in the fridge and then either eaten cold or reheated. In fact, in an experiment for the BBC programme *Trust Me, I'm a Doctor* in 2014, reheating pre-cooked and chilled pasta was found to double the amount of resistant starch it contained. Then in 2015, researchers at the College of Chemical Sciences in Sri Lanka found the same thing happens when you reheat rice. Eating bread that's been frozen then defrosted has the same effect. But research by the US Potato Board in 2013 found that potatoes are different – eating them chilled (as in potato salad) gives you the most resistant starch.

Safety reminder: If using rice, make sure it's cooled and chilled quickly and reheat it only once within 24 hours to avoid the risk of food poisoning.

How coffee, tea, red wine and dark chocolate can boost your biome

The good news is you can enjoy coffee, tea, wine and dark chocolate as part of a healthy, gut-friendly diet – though in moderation, of course!

All of these foods and drinks contain polyphenols. Polyphenols are plant chemicals that can benefit health. Only a small number of polyphenols are absorbed in the small intestine – the rest go to the large intestine, where they act like a prebiotic, increasing numbers of health-boosting bacteria in the gut, such as *Bacteroidetes*, *Lactobacilli* and *Bifidobacteria*. Not only do polyphenols boost levels of beneficial bacteria, they also stop the growth of harmful bacteria such as *Clostridium*. Fruit and vegetables also contain polyphenols, but not in as high concentrations. So it's good to know that you can indulge in that cappuccino (without sugar), glass of red wine or chunk of dark chocolate with a clear conscience!

But there is a caveat – to get these health benefits without any negative effects, you need to enjoy these drinks and foods in moderation.

Coffee

Drinking coffee has been shown to boost mood and extend your life by preventing cardiovascular disease, Alzheimer's, gallstones and certain cancers. Recent research suggests this could at least in part be down to the beneficial effect it has on gut bacteria. Studies, including one at the University of Groningen in the Netherlands in 2016, have found that people who drink coffee have a more diverse biome, with more of the good bacteria.

In 2007 food scientists at the Spanish National Research Council in Madrid found that as well as polyphenols, coffee contains soluble fibre. A study at the Nestlé Research Centre in Switzerland in 2009 backed these findings when it showed that beneficial gut bacteria such as *Bifidobacteria* can easily digest the fibre in coffee and in the process they make the gut-friendly short-chain fatty acids butyrate and acetic acid.

Tea
Green tea and black tea both have a similar amount of polyphenols, but different types. They are both made from the leaves of the *Camellia sinensis* plant, so they start out with the same type of polyphenols – known as flavonoids. Green tea is made by steaming and drying the leaves. To make black tea, the leaves are left to ferment. During fermentation the flavonoids change. As a result, black tea finishes up with different flavonoids to those in green tea.

But beware of too much caffeine
Despite the health benefits of tea and coffee, moderation is key as coffee and tea both contain caffeine. Too much caffeine can cause several problems in the gut. It can increase the amount of acid in your stomach, which can give you an upset stomach or cause heartburn. Caffeine also triggers peristalsis in the gut, which is great if you suffer from constipation, but if not it can cause diarrhoea. Excess caffeine can also aggravate IBS.

Too much caffeine also raises levels of the stress hormone cortisol, which can cause anxiety and insomnia – this can have a knock-on negative effect on gut bacteria.

The amount of caffeine in tea and coffee can vary quite widely and depends on factors like the brand, how much coffee/tea is used and how long it is left to brew.

Happy gut tip

If you suffer from anaemia, avoid drinking tea with a meal. Wait until about half an hour afterwards. Tannins – one of the polyphenols in green and black teas – can hamper absorption of non-haem iron found in plant-based foods such as dark green vegetables, wholegrains, peas and dried fruit. Non-haem iron is much harder for your body to absorb than haem iron which is found in meat, poultry and seafood.

Kombucha
This is a fermented black or green tea. It's naturally fizzy with a slightly vinegary taste and is full of beneficial bacteria. You make it by adding a bacteria and yeast culture (called a scoby) to tea and sugar and leaving it to ferment. If you want to make your own you'll find a recipe in **Chapter 13**.

Dark chocolate
While it's great news for chocoholics that dark chocolate is rich in polyphenols and contains less sugar and fat than milk chocolate, it still contains quite high levels. For example, a well-known brand of 70 per cent dark chocolate contains almost 30 per cent sugar and just over 40 per cent fat! So enjoy dark chocolate in moderation. Drinking unsweetened cocoa is the healthiest way to get your chocolate fix, as you get the benefit of the polyphenols without the added sugar and fat. Cocoa and chocolate also contain caffeine.

How much caffeine should I have?

It's hard to say how much caffeine is too much, as sensitivity to it varies from one person to another. But in 2015 the European Food Safety Authority (EFSA) recommended a safe daily limit of 400 mg for adults. This is roughly the equivalent of four medium strength mugs of tea or four cups of ground coffee, depending on the strength of the brew.

Caffeine content of drinks/foods

Drink/food	Caffeine content (approx.)
Tea (mug)	55 mg–140 mg
Instant coffee (cup)	54 mg
Ground coffee (cup)	105 mg
Cocoa (cup)	5 mg
50 g plain chocolate	Up to 50 mg
50 g milk chocolate	25 mg

The good news is that decaffeinated coffee also contains prebiotic fibre, so you can drink it in place of normal coffee once you've reached your daily healthy limit and your gut will still benefit.

Enjoy a tipple

Having the odd tipple could also boost your gut health. Dutch researchers also found that drinking a glass of wine can help people maintain their levels of good gut bacteria.

Like coffee and tea, wine contains polyphenols. Resveratrol is the main polyphenol found in wine. Wine has soluble sugars called polysaccharides too, which are also prebiotic. Red wines seem the most beneficial, as they have up to five times more prebiotics than white. Research shows that red wine boosts levels of *Bacteroidetes* which is linked to being a healthy weight, as well as *Bifidobacterium* and *Lactobacillus*. The *American Gut*, a project set up at the University of California, San Diego in 2012 to research the effects people's lifestyles have on their biome, found that people who had at least one alcoholic drink a week had more diverse microflora than teetotallers.

But drink in moderation

But as with coffee and tea, moderation is vital, as too much alcohol makes your stomach produce more acid than normal which can damage the gut lining. The excess acid can also cause reflux – which is where stomach acids travel up into the throat and cause damage.

Drinking a lot of alcohol can also make it harder to digest food and absorb nutrients, especially proteins and vitamins. This is because alcohol reduces the amount of digestive enzymes the pancreas produces to help us to break down fats and carbohydrates. Drinking too much can also cause stomach pain and diarrhoea.

Another reason why you should keep an eye on your alcohol intake is because it contains sugar. Dry wines and ciders and lagers, beers, stouts and spirits contain the least sugar while, as you would expect, sweet wines,

THE HAPPY GUT GUIDE

ciders, cocktails and liqueurs contain the most. For example, a medium (175 ml) glass of dry white wine contains around half a teaspoon of sugar while a 50-ml measure of Baileys Irish Cream contains two teaspoons. While spirits are low in sugar, mixers are not. A 250-ml can of gin and tonic contains 3.5 teaspoons of sugar.

You can lessen the effects of alcohol on your stomach by eating before or while you drink, as this slows down the rate at which your body absorbs alcohol. Alternating alcoholic drinks with non-alcoholic (preferably sugar-free) ones can also help you keep your drinking in check.

Alcohol guidelines for men and women

Drinkaware states that to keep health risks from alcohol at a low level it is safest not to regularly drink more than 14 units a week. This is equal to six medium (175 ml) glasses of wine (13 per cent alcohol) or six pints of beer/lager (4 per cent alcohol) per week. For more information visit **www.drinkaware.co.uk**.

Beneficial bug checker

Below is a handy checklist of the main beneficial gut bacteria, how they improve your health and which foods and drinks will boost your levels.

Bacteria type	Health benefits	Foods/drinks that boost levels
Akkermansia	Strengthen gut wall, anti-inflammatory, curb weight gain	Fruit, vegetables, tea, coffee, red wine
Bacteroidetes	Strengthen gut wall, anti-inflammatory, curb weight gain	Fruit, vegetables and pulses
Bifidobacterium	Protect gut from 'bad' microbes, help ease IBS	Natural yogurt, cheese and kefir and pickled vegetables
Lactobacillus	Protect gut from 'bad' bugs, boost mood, prevent weight gain	Natural yogurt, cheese, kefir
Streptococcus thermophilus	Anti-inflammatory, aid lactose digestion	Certain natural yogurts and cheeses and kefir

10 herbs and spices for a happy gut

Herbs and spices are rich in gut-friendly polyphenols and inulin. Many of them also help improve digestion and ease tummy problems.

1. Black pepper

Black pepper has long been used in Ayurvedic (traditional Indian) medicine to ease stomach problems. Indian researchers claim that adding black pepper to your meals improves digestion and reduces bloating. It may also help your body break down fats.

The key ingredient is piperine, which encourages the release of hydrochloric acid and digestive enzymes. Grinding whole black peppercorns gives the most flavour.

2. Camomile

Camomile is said to ease cramps and bloating by relaxing the muscles in the gastrointestinal tract. It's also a relaxing herb, making it very useful for treating stress-related IBS. It contains the amino acid glycine, a muscle and nerve relaxant. Camomile teabags are widely available in supermarkets. Alternatively, you can grow camomile in your garden and make your own infusion from the fresh or dried flower heads.

Note

Camomile is generally safe, but avoid taking it if you have an allergy to the *Asteraceae* (*Compositae*) family of plants, which includes aster, chrysanthemum, mugwort, ragweed and ragwort.

3. Caraway seeds
The ancient Greeks used caraway seeds to help digestion. They are thought to stimulate the production of gastric juices and contain a natural antibiotic. The volatile oils and other chemicals in caraway help relax muscle spasms in the intestines and release trapped wind. You can make a caraway infusion by adding one cup of boiling water to one teaspoon of seeds. Leave to infuse for about 10 minutes, strain and drink.

4. Cardamom
The cardamom plant is native to South East Asia, Sri Lanka and southern India and is often used in Indian cookery. Cardamom features in Ayurvedic and Chinese medicine as an anti-flatulent and indigestion aid. It's said to relieve wind by easing spasms in the intestines and helping fat digestion by encouraging the release of bile. The whole pods can be chewed, or you can add them to curries and desserts.

5. Coriander
Both Ayurvedic and Chinese medicine use coriander for counteracting indigestion, bloating, diarrhoea and nausea as well as protecting against food poisoning. Coriander seeds have a laxative effect. Add the chopped leaves to curries and other savoury dishes after cooking, or add boiling water to a few fresh leaves and brew for 5 minutes before drinking.

6. Dill seeds
Dill seed oil is the main ingredient of gripe water, which relieves colic in babies by breaking down trapped wind and easing tummy cramps and spasms. Dill seeds are just as effective for digestive problems in adults.

You can easily grow your own plants from seed, either outdoors or indoors. Once the seeds turn brown, hang the seed heads upside down in a paper bag for a couple of weeks. Once they're dry, the seeds will fall into the bag, ready for you to store them in an airtight jar.

To make a dill seed infusion, leave one to two teaspoons of dried seeds in a cup of boiling water for about 10 minutes, then strain and drink.

7. Fennel

Both the plant and the seeds have long been used to ease stomach cramps and wind. The active ingredient are terpenoids, which have a carminative (wind-relieving) effect. Fennel also stimulates the release of bile, which means it may help break down fats in food. In *The Complete German Commission E Monographs* – a guide written by the German Commission E that reviews herbal drugs and preparations from medicinal plants for their quality, safety and effectiveness – the recommended dose is one to one-and-a-half teaspoons of seeds a day.

The seeds taste like aniseed and are quite pleasant to chew or, if you prefer, you can make an infusion using one teaspoon per cup of boiling water. Leave to brew for 10–15 minutes, then strain and drink. Fennel can be eaten raw, finely sliced in salads, or roasted in a little olive oil and served with fish or chicken.

Warning
Avoid fennel if you have epilepsy as it could induce a seizure.

8. Ginger

Ginger root has traditionally been used to ease nausea and other digestive problems in Ayurvedic, Chinese and herbal medicine. It's thought to stimulate digestion and tone the digestive tract muscles, which helps food pass through the system more easily, causing less irritation to the intestinal walls. Ginger also contains zingibain, an enzyme that helps the body break down food and absorb nutrients.

It's cheap and widely available, and can be added to savoury dishes such as stir-fries and curries. You can make a ginger infusion by grating a 2.5-cm cube into a cup and adding boiling water. Leave to brew for 5 minutes, then strain and, if desired, sweeten with honey to taste. Alternatively, sprinkle a third of a teaspoon of dried ginger into a cup of ordinary tea, or eat one or two pieces of crystallised ginger.

9. Peppermint

Peppermint, used by the ancient Greeks for gut problems, is great for relieving indigestion and flatulence. It is good for IBS sufferers, as it eases gut spasms. In 2008, the *British Medical Journal* (*BMJ*) reported that almost half of IBS sufferers found relief from their symptoms when they took peppermint oil. Its active ingredients are menthol, menthone and eucalyptol which relax the intestinal muscles.

You can take peppermint in an infusion, oil, herb or capsule form. Peppermint teabags are readily available in supermarkets, or you can add a few drops of peppermint oil to half a tumbler of warm water. You can also grow your own mint in the garden and use it in cooking or to make an infusion. Simply pour boiling water over 30 g (two tablespoons) of the fresh herb and leave to brew for 5–10 minutes. Then strain and serve.

Some people argue the enteric-coated capsules work best because they protect the active ingredients from stomach acids and are absorbed in the intestines, where they are most needed.

10. Turmeric

Turmeric is anti-inflammatory and is thought to prevent the growth of 'bad' bacteria in the gut. It also helps calm gut spasms and diarrhoea and relieves wind and bloating, so it's recommended for IBS. It also helps with digestion because it stimulates the release of bile.

Medicinal charcoal

Charcoal is an old-fashioned remedy for treating excess stomach and intestinal wind. The charcoal absorbs the excess gas in the gut. You can buy medicinal charcoal in biscuit, capsule, tablet or powder form from health food shops, pharmacies and online (see **Resources**). Charcoal is safe to take during pregnancy and breastfeeding.

Eat mindfully

It's not just *what* you eat but *how* you eat that can affect your gut health. With the fast pace of modern life, it's easy to rush your food – perhaps even eating while on the move, rather than sitting down at the table and taking the time to enjoy it. Eating too fast prevents your gut from digesting your food properly. Not taking time to relax when you're eating can cause indigestion and other problems. It takes your brain about 20 minutes to send out signals to your stomach that you are full, so if you eat too quickly you may well eat more than you need, which over time will lead to weight gain.

Chewing your food well will give the enzymes in your saliva more time to start breaking down your food, and to stimulate your gastric juices. Taking a slow and mindful approach will improve your digestion and help you avoid eating too much and suffering from wind and bloating.

Happy gut tip

Eat three proper meals a day with gaps in between, rather than constantly grazing. Have at least 12 hours without food overnight. Research shows that giving your gut some downtime boosts the health of the biome and enables gut-strengthening bugs like *Akkermansia* to thrive and do their job.

More good eating habits

- Eat at regular times to help your digestive system to settle into a routine.

- Avoid eating large meals, as overeating can cause bloating and diarrhoea.

- Eat slowly – if you gobble your food down quickly you're likely to swallow air and suffer from wind and bloating.

- Chew your food well – up to 30 times – to give enzymes in your saliva more time to start breaking it down and to stimulate gastric juices.

- Chewing too fast means your stomach and intestines have to cope with large pieces of food which can cause digestive problems.

- Drink plenty of fluids, especially water – this combines with fibre in the intestine to make your stools bulkier and easier to pass, and it rehydrates you if you have diarrhoea.

- Don't eat when you're feeling stressed, or while you're on the move. If you can, wait until you can sit down and relax.

- Sit still for at least a few minutes after a meal. Getting up and rushing around deprives your gut of the oxygen it needs to digest food, and can cause indigestion, stomach cramps and bloating.

Is chewing gum good for digestion?

The short answer is probably not. When you chew gum you may swallow excess air, which can cause bloating and tummy pain. Also, when you chew you send your gut signals that it's about to receive food, so enzymes and acids are released but without the food they're intended to digest. This can cause bloating and an overproduction of stomach acid. You may also start having problems producing enzymes and stomach acids when you actually do eat food. The artificial sweeteners in sugar-free gum can also cause gastrointestinal symptoms such as bloating and diarrhoea in some people.

In a nutshell: foods and drinks for a happy gut

- Fermented foods for their friendly flora, like full-fat natural yogurt, kefir, certain cheeses and sauerkraut.

- Lots of different coloured fruit and vegetables to feed and increase your numbers of beneficial bugs.

- Green bananas and chilled or chilled-and-reheated pasta, rice and potatoes for gut-friendly resistant starch.

- Moderate amounts of tea, coffee, wine and dark chocolate for probiotic-promoting polyphenols.

- Herbs and spices like peppermint, ginger and turmeric to ease digestive problems.

CHAPTER 8

SLEEP YOUR
GUT HEALTHY

Most of us are aware that we need to get the right amount of good quality sleep to function well both mentally and physically. In a poll of 8,250 people in 2017, researchers at Oxford Economics and the National Centre for Social Research (NatCen) found that getting regular sound sleep was the biggest indicator of well-being. But did you know that plenty of sleep is also vital for a healthy gut and vice versa? Insomnia is linked to tiredness, lack of energy, difficulty concentrating and irritability, as well as weight gain, type 2 diabetes and low mood. It seems that all of these conditions may be linked to the type of bacteria we have in our gut. In this chapter we look at the relationship between the gut, sleep and our general well-being and what steps you can take to get more shut-eye.

Sleep deprivation and weight gain

In **Chapter 1** we talked about how certain gut bacteria, such as *Firmicutes,* were linked with weight gain. Now a 2017 study at the Biomedical Centre at Uppsala University, Sweden has found that not getting enough sleep for just two nights cuts certain beneficial bacteria by half. Participants were also less sensitive to insulin after two nights of sleep deprivation, and they had more *Firmicutes* and other bacteria linked with weight gain. This is probably because feeling tired makes you more likely to want to eat the sugary, refined, fatty snacks that give you a quick energy boost and that *Firmicutes* like to feed on. Lots of other research shows that getting plenty of sleep helps you keep your weight in check.

Sleep deficit and diabetes

A lack of sleep is also linked with the body being less sensitive to insulin, which means the body has to produce more and more of it to keep blood sugar levels steady. This can eventually lead to weight gain and type 2 diabetes.

Lack of sleep and leaky gut

Going short of sleep causes stress that leads to higher cortisol levels, which have been linked to leaky gut syndrome. Remember, this is where undigested food particles, bacteria, toxins and germs leak into the bloodstream, causing inflammation and various health issues. Also, the body repairs itself during the deep sleep phase of the sleep cycle. So a lack of good-quality sleep means the body doesn't get enough time to repair the gut lining, again raising the risk of developing a leaky gut.

How the biome affects sleep

A 2016 study by scientists at the University of Zaragoza, Spain, suggested that not only does the quality of our sleep affect our biome, but it in turn affects our sleep. They found that microbes living in our gut activate a protein called TLR2 in the intestines. TLR2 helps transport serotonin – the 'happy hormone' involved in sleep, mood and appetite – around the body. They claimed that having the 'wrong' types of microbes in the gut led to less serotonin being carried around the body. Low serotonin levels are linked to sleep problems, depression and being overweight.

How much sleep do I need?

Sleep experts say that the idea that 8 hours' sleep is the norm for healthy adults is a myth and that the average amount of sleep an adult needs is probably nearer to between 7 and 7½ hours.

But individual sleep needs can vary quite widely, with some people being able to function well on as little as 4 hours' sleep. Age is another factor – babies need up to 18 hours' sleep a day while teenagers need around nine.

Listen to your body

So it seems that everyone is different and the answer can be found by listening to your own body. If you can fall asleep fairly quickly at night when tired, enjoy mostly unbroken sleep and wake up feeling refreshed and alert, then you're probably getting sufficient sleep. On the other hand, if you often have trouble going to sleep, have broken sleep and wake up the next day feeling groggy and exhausted, you can assume you're not sleeping enough.

So what can you do to help ensure you get the right amount of good quality sleep? Clearly, following the advice in this book is a good start, as it will help ensure you have a healthy biome, which will in turn help improve your sleep. Below are more top tips to help you sleep more soundly:

1. Get outdoors in daylight

Get outdoors in daylight to stop production of the sleep-promoting hormone melatonin. This encourages your body to release it sooner at night, making it easier for you to drop off at bedtime and to sleep more deeply. Blue light, which is light from a blue sky on a clear day, is thought to be the most beneficial.

2. Eat tryptophan-rich foods

Eat foods rich in tryptophan, the amino acid your gut bacteria use to produce serotonin, which is converted into melatonin at night. Tryptophan-rich foods include dairy foods, chicken, turkey, salmon, bananas, dates, rice, oats, wholegrain breads and cereals. Ensure you're neither too hungry nor too full at bedtime, as both can cause wakefulness.

3. Eat more fibre

We've already talked about how fibre can boost your good gut bacteria and improve your general health, but now recent research suggests it can help improve your sleep. It seems a diet high in fibre and low in sugar and saturated fats cuts the time it takes to fall asleep and improves sleep quality. This is likely down to these foods boosting the number of beneficial bugs linked with better sleep.

4. Curtail the coffee

How quickly you metabolise caffeine varies from one person to another. If you're a fast metaboliser you can probably get away with drinking coffee or cola any time of day or night. But if you find you have problems dropping off after having coffee or cola at night, it's likely you are a slow metaboliser and will sleep better if you avoid drinking them, or eating chocolate, after 2 p.m. While tea has around half as much caffeine – about 50 mg per cup – it's advisable not to drink it near bedtime if you have sleep problems. Redbush (rooibos) tea, decaffeinated tea or coffee, or herbal teas (which are caffeine-free) make good alternatives.

Happy gut tip

Chicory coffee is not only a good caffeine-free alternative to coffee, it also contains inulin – a type of fibre that boosts good microbes.

5. Get active

Exercise during the day to raise your body temperature and metabolism. They will drop a few hours later, signalling to your brain it's time for sleep. Avoid exercising after 8 p.m. otherwise your body temperature could still be raised at bedtime, and keep you awake. Being inactive is linked to difficulty dropping off and restlessness. Exercise also helps you to de-stress, and stress is linked to insomnia.

6. Relax and unwind

Make time to relax and unwind before bedtime. Devise your own evening ritual that enables you to 'put the day to bed'. This might involve watching TV – if you find it relaxing – but avoid watching anything that could prey on your mind later on when you're trying to go to sleep. Alternatively, try reading or listening to relaxing music.

7. Dim the lights

Dim or turn off the lights 2 hours before bed. Darkness triggers melatonin production.

8. Take a warm bath/shower

Your temperature rises with the warmth and then falls – helping you to drop off. The warmth also eases muscular and mental tension, especially if you sprinkle a few drops of relaxing essential oils like lavender or camomile into your bath or onto your shower sponge. Or add Epsom salts to your bath – they contain magnesium, dubbed 'nature's own tranquiliser', which relaxes both mind and muscles.

9. Avoid alcohol at bedtime

It might help you relax and drop off more quickly, but it's a stimulant, so it can make you wake up during the night. It's also a diuretic, so you're more likely to wake up to go to the loo in the night.

10. Make your bedroom sleep-friendly

Make your bedroom as cosy and inviting as you can to make bedtime a pleasure. Choose relaxing shades such as pale green or blue for the walls, bedding and curtains.

- **Keep your bedroom at around 16°C** – your brain tries to lower your body temperature at night to slow down your metabolism and aid sleep.

- **Hang dark, heavy curtains and black-out blinds** – darkness prompts the pineal gland in the brain to make melatonin. Light shining through the bedroom window has the opposite effect.

- **Check your mattress gives you the right level of support.** Lie on your back and slip a hand under your lower back. You should be able to fit your hand in the gap between your back and the mattress. If there's no space, the mattress is too soft. A bed board under the mattress could help. If there is a lot of room, the mattress is too hard for you. If you're not planning to buy a new mattress soon, a mattress topper – the cheaper alternative – might help.

- **Pick a pillow that keeps your spine level with your neck.** The best pillow thickness for you depends on your shoulder width – if they're narrow, choose a flatter pillow; if you have broad shoulders, you might even need two pillows.

- **Banish TVs, computers, tablets and smartphones from your bedroom** – so you associate it with sleep and sex only.

- **Turn off technology.** Using technology last thing at night can overstimulate your brain, leaving you 'tired but wired' so you can't switch off and fall asleep. The bright light they emit can also stop your brain producing melatonin. Log off computers, tablets and smartphones at least 2 hours before bed. If watching TV helps you relax, choose something 'light' that won't overstimulate your brain.

- **Tip:** If you like to use the alarm on your smartphone put it on airplane mode before bed, so it doesn't buzz through the night with notifications and wake you.

11. Inhale lavender

Sprinkle a few drops of soothing lavender oil on your pillow at night. Inhaling lavender oil at night has been shown to be as effective for treating insomnia as taking commonly prescribed sleeping tablets, helping to improve sleep quality by 20 per cent. Research suggests lavender increases slow-wave sleep, the very deep sleep phase in which the heartbeat slows and muscles relax. Using lavender oil during the day could also help you improve your sleep by helping you to manage stress. In 2012, researchers at Eulji University, South Korea found that sniffing lavender oil for 5 minutes daily lowers levels of the stress hormone cortisol. Rosemary oil was also found to be an effective stress-reliever.

12. Take a relaxing herb

Take a herbal supplement or tea containing one or more of these sedating herbs – valerian, hops, camomile, lemon balm or passiflora – to help you drop off more easily and sleep more deeply.

13. Go to bed when drowsy

Only go to bed when you feel drowsy. If you can't fall asleep after about 20 minutes, get up and do something you find relaxing, like reading or listening to soothing music. Or make yourself a glass of warm milk with a sprinkle of nutmeg. The calcium in the milk and the nutmeg have relaxing properties that will help you drop off when you return to bed. Only return to bed when you feel sleepy, to help your brain associate your bed with sleep.

14. Write down your woes

If you have a tendency to lie awake mulling over problems or thinking about your activities the next day, try clearing your mind by jotting down any worries, or a brief plan for the day ahead, before you go to bed.

   If you wake up during the night and start thinking about problems, try telling yourself firmly: 'You can't resolve this now, so go to sleep and think about it tomorrow.'

15. Manage stress

If jotting down your concerns before bed doesn't stop you from lying awake worrying, you may be suffering from excessive stress. In the next chapter you'll find lots of tips to help you manage your stress levels and enjoy better sleep and gut health.

In a nutshell: why you need good quality sleep and how to get it

- Sleep needs vary but the average adult needs 7 to 7½ hours a night.
- A lack of sleep can damage the gut and cause weight gain, type 2 diabetes and depression.
- You can improve your sleep by boosting beneficial gut bugs, exercising in daylight, winding down before bed and avoiding late-night technology.

CHAPTER 9

DIAL DOWN STRESS

Stress is what you feel when you are under more pressure than you are able to handle. We all have our own personal threshold – one person may cope well in a situation that another might find stressful. It's all down to each person's perception of it and their ability to deal with it.

When you feel stressed your body produces the stress hormones cortisol, noradrenaline and adrenaline to help you cope. This is the 'fight-or-flight' response that is a short-term reaction to a stressful situation, such as fighting off an aggressive neighbour or fleeing from a dangerous animal, which enabled our ancestors to either fight against a threat or run away from it.

Nowadays we are more likely to face constant stresses in our daily lives and long-term exposure to stress hormones can have a bad effect on our gut and overall health. This chapter explains the signs of stress, how it can affect your gut and how your gut can affect the way you deal with stress.

Take the stress test

Your body may be telling you you're stressed without you even realising it. Answer the questions below to find out if you're stressed.

1. Do you constantly crave chocolate, sweets, breads, cakes, caffeine or alcohol?

2. Are you a bit plump around your middle?

3. Do you wolf down your food and suffer from wind and bloating afterwards?

4. Do you have frequent bouts of IBS?

5. Do you have frequent headaches or migraines?

6. Do you suffer from muscular aches and pains in the shoulders, neck or back?

7. Do you have difficulty falling asleep or staying asleep?

8. Do you have any of these nervous habits – nail biting, hair pulling, fist clenching, foot tapping, teeth grinding, blinking or nervous tics?

9. Do you suffer from hair loss?

10. Do you find it hard to concentrate?

11. Are you forgetful?

12. Do you suffer from pre-menstrual syndrome (PMS)?

13. Do you often feel tense or anxious?

14. Do you suffer from low mood?

15. Do you have panic attacks?

16. Are you often irritable?

17. Do you often fly off the handle for no good reason?

18. Do you get frequent flare-ups of skin conditions like eczema, acne or psoriasis?

19. Do you suffer from allergies or food intolerances?

20. Do you have frequent asthma attacks?

If you answered 'yes' to two or more questions it's likely you're suffering the effects of stress. The more times you answered 'yes' the more stressed you're likely to be. Many of these symptoms may be linked to stress hormones like cortisol and adrenaline affecting the balance between your good and bad bacteria.

How stress affects your biome

Research suggests that during the stress response, cortisol and adrenaline can wipe out a large proportion of your good gut bacteria. A 2008 study at the University of Technology Sydney found that during exam week, university students had less *Lactobacilli* in their gut than when they started the semester. This reduction in good bacteria might help explain why we tend to suffer from more health problems when we're stressed.

Now read on to find out more about how stress can affect your gut health and how that can have a knock-on effect on your general well-being.

Gut reaction

One of the reasons stress affects the gut is because the brain and gut are linked by the enteric nervous system, which controls the gut and enables the brain and gut to constantly exchange messages. This means that whatever affects the brain is likely to affect the gut, and vice versa. This explains why a stressful situation, like taking an exam or losing a loved one, can make some people feel sick or lose their appetite. Scientists use the term gut-brain to describe this close relationship between the brain and the gut. So if you take steps to deal with stress you will not only calm your mind, but your gut as well.

Stress and weight gain

When we're stressed we naturally crave sweet and starchy foods for a quick energy boost. As we've already seen, these foods have a bad effect on the biome and lead to fat being stored around the middle. Also, stress hormones boost blood sugar levels, to give us energy for either 'fight or flight'. If we don't burn off the energy through exercise the excess sugar is stored as fat around the middle in readiness for the next stressful situation. Belly fat breaks down into fatty acids more easily, which can then be sent to the liver to be turned into energy quickly. We've already discussed the links between belly fat, insulin resistance and type 2 diabetes in **Chapter 1**.

Stress and gut pain

Stress hormones can trigger gut pain. This is because, as well as adrenaline, the body produces a hormone called CRF (corticotropin-releasing factor) which triggers the release of cortisol. It's thought when a person suffers from prolonged stress, adrenaline and CRF affect the nerve cells in the gut, making them more sensitive to pain, so that even normal gut contractions are very painful. This could explain the tummy pain many people experience when they are stressed.

Other ways stress can cause bloating and pain

Also, if you eat when you feel tense you may swallow excess air which then causes bloating and pain in the gut. Some people 'over-breathe' when they're anxious. Air then travels down the gullet into the stomach where it gets trapped, causing bloating and pain.

Stress can affect digestion

A rushed, stressful lifestyle often means that people don't take the time to go to the loo when they need to, which can make the bowel 'lazy' and prone to constipation.

Stress hormones can also affect how quickly food is pushed through your gut. With some people digestion slows down, causing constipation, while in others it can speed up, causing diarrhoea. Constipation cuts the number and types of friendly bacteria in the gut and boosts the growth of less helpful ones.

Stress and leaky gut syndrome

Other experts say that, over time, stress hormones like adrenaline and cortisol irritate the gut lining, making it hypersensitive and prone to leaky gut syndrome. This is where the gut wall is weakened and lets partly digested food leak through into the bloodstream, where it causes inflammation, allergies, food intolerances and skin problems.

Stress and sleep

In the previous chapter we saw how sleep problems can cause stress and stress can cause sleep problems, which can lead to a vicious cycle. Not only that, a lack of sleep makes us more likely to crave sugary or refined, starchy foods for a quick energy boost and drink too much alcohol, which in turn negatively affects our biome.

So, stress has a knock-on negative effect on various aspects of our health, including our gut health, which in turn affects our general mental and physical well-being. Clearly, managing stress is essential for a happy gut and overall good health. But that's only part of the picture. It seems that when your biome has the right balance of beneficial bacteria, it helps you to cope better with stress and reduces the effects of stress on the body.

Beat stress with beneficial bugs

Beneficial bugs like *Bifidobacteria, Lactobacilli* or *Bacteroidetes* make the 'happy hormone' serotonin, which helps you to stay positive in stressful times. They also lower cortisol levels so that stress has fewer negative effects on the body. So it seems the connection between stress and the gut biome works both ways – stress can affect the bacteria and they in turn can affect our response to stress.

So, to beat stress you need to both look after your biome by following the diet and lifestyle advice in this book and take practical steps to cut stress in your daily life and counteract its harmful effects.

Dial down stress: say 'no' to overload

When you're feeling overwhelmed by having too much to do at home or at work, step back for a moment and:

1. **Prioritise** – what are the most important tasks that need doing as soon as possible and what can be left until later?

2. **Delegate** – instead of trying to do everything yourself, identify tasks you can pass on to someone else.

3. **Ditch** – non-essential tasks you don't have time to do.

Tell yourself everything is OK

Our survival instinct means our brains are programmed to be on guard in case something bad happens, which can make us feel anxious. When you find yourself worrying unnecessarily about the future, try telling yourself: 'Everything is OK right now.' This will help to calm your fears and encourage you to focus on the present.

Spend time with family and friends

Having a good social network has been shown to help people deal better with stressful events such as job loss, divorce and bereavement. Talking over problems with someone you trust can help you get things into perspective and find ways to resolve issues.

Make time for me-time

Taking time out for yourself every day – even for just a few minutes – is a great stress-reliever. Find a space where you can be alone and undisturbed and do whatever helps you escape the stresses and strains of modern life. When you get home, get out of work mode by changing your clothes. Light an aromatherapy candle and breathe in the scent. Read a newspaper or a novel, watch your favourite TV programme or soak in a hot bath – anything that helps you unwind. A little bit of time alone has been shown to lower stress hormones and boost mood and memory. Making 'me-time' a daily habit no matter how busy you are will help you to keep your stress levels in check.

Appreciate the simple things in life

Every night before bed think of at least one pleasurable thing you experienced that day. It doesn't have to be anything major – a 2017 poll of 2,000 Britons found that it's the simple pleasures in life that make people happy, such as sharing a kiss or a hug with a loved one, snuggling into freshly laundered bedding, soaking in a hot bath or enjoying a belly laugh with friends. Enjoying and appreciating the simple things in life, rather than focusing on the material goods you don't have, helps you to feel happier, more relaxed and less stressed.

Find the positive in a negative

Having a more positive outlook on life can help you avoid feeling stressed, even when things go wrong. When bad things happen, it's not the event itself that makes you feel stressed, but how you perceive it. So, for example, if you attend a job interview and don't get the job, instead of telling yourself 'I'm a complete failure', try to view it more positively, as in: 'I didn't get the job but my application impressed them enough for them to want to interview me and it was good practice for the next time, when I could be successful.'

Beat workplace stress

Stress is now the most common reason for British workers to be signed off on long-term sick leave – ahead of back problems, stroke, heart attack, cancer and mental-health issues – and work itself can be a major cause of stress. A report by the Chartered Institute of Personnel and Development in 2011 blamed job insecurity caused by the economic downturn, an excessive workload, poor management and restructuring in the workplace for work-related stress. The main causes of work-related stress are:

- Lack of control over your work situation
- Working long hours, or working shifts
- Not having time for breaks
- Having too heavy a workload, or too much responsibility
- Lack of help and support from your co-workers or supervisors
- Concerns about job security
- A lack of opportunities to advance
- Doing a job that is boring and repetitive

Many people are working longer and longer hours, often without breaks, in the hope of impressing their managers and holding on to their jobs.

Unfortunately, working in this way is likely to make you more stressed, which could hamper your performance and make you more prone to illness – this would likely make you less, rather than more, productive. Below are ten top tips to help make your working day less stressful:

1. Get ready for work

Prepare for work the night before by getting your clothes and any work equipment ready. If you have problems deciding what to wear, try having a specific outfit for each day of the week (depending on the season), so that you don't have to think about it. Plan your breakfast and prepare your packed lunch to save time in the morning.

2. Adjust your workspace

Adjust your workspace to help you sit upright and avoid tension in the neck, shoulders and lower back. If you work with a computer screen it should be straight in front of you, so you don't need to twist your neck or shoulders. You should be able to see your screen sitting upright, not leaning backwards or forwards. The top of the screen should be at the same level as your eyes.

Your seat should be adjusted so that your upper arms are at your sides and your wrists and forearms are horizontal when you use your keyboard. Your pelvis should be slightly higher than your knees. Your feet should rest flat on the floor. If you can't manage that, use a shallow footrest. If you're unsure if your workspace suits your needs, ask your employer to check that it complies with health and safety regulations.

3. Go green

Having a plant on your desk at work could cut your stress levels, lower your blood pressure and improve your productivity. These benefits are thought to be down to the calming influence of nature and the air-purifying and humidifying effects of plants. Foliage plants such as palms, ferns, spider plants, weeping figs and rubber plants are thought to work best. They absorb the harmful chemicals and pollutants computers and office furnishings give off and put moisture and oxygen back into the air.

4. Declutter your desk

A cluttered desk can make work more stressful. Piles of paperwork sitting on your desk can be overwhelming and searching through them for the documents you need is time-consuming. Decluttering your desk makes it easier to focus on the task in hand. Sort through paperwork and either in-tray it, file it or bin it. If it you need to act on it, put it in your in-tray to deal with as soon as possible. If you will need it sometime in the future, file it away where you can find it easily. If it is out of date, or no longer needed, bin it.

Tip: Get in the habit of tidying your desk every night before you leave, so that you are greeted with an organised workspace next day.

5. Organise your workload

Write a to-do list at the end of every working day, ready for the next day. If you have a long to-do list, number tasks in terms of urgency and importance, then do them in that order. Crossing off tasks as soon as you complete them will help you feel in control and that you are making progress.

If you have several telephone calls to make, letters to write and emails to respond to, try 'chunking' to save time. That means making all your telephone calls in one go, then writing all of your letters and then your emails.

6. Stop for a chat

Although too many interruptions from emails, phone calls, text messages and colleagues chatting can lead to work piling up, being sociable at work has been shown to cut stress. So take 5 minutes for a cuppa and a chat, if you can, during your working day.

7. Avoid second-hand stress

Stress in the workplace can be contagious – if a colleague is stressed you can unconsciously pick up their negative vibes. To avoid 'catching' stress when a colleague is complaining about their work or personal life, try to say something positive about their situation or offer to help them. If they keep on being negative, try taking a break – perhaps by going to make a cup of tea. If you can't walk away, make a conscious effort to stay positive and avoid adopting their mindset.

8. Take a break

No matter how busy you are, you should make time for one or two short breaks during your working day. Going for a walk or even just reading a newspaper – preferably away from your desk – can take your mind off work and lower your stress levels. Don't worry about wasting valuable working time – taking a break has been shown to boost productivity.

9. 'Desk-ercise'

Stretching your body every hour or two stops muscular tension from developing and gets the blood flowing, helping you avoid blood clots. Even just walking to the kitchen or going to the photocopier can help. A 2017 study at the University of Leicester found that 5 minutes of arm exercises every half hour reduced the risk of type 2 diabetes. So if you don't have time to leave your desk, try these 'desk-ercises' from your chair:

- Tighten your calf and thigh muscles, hold then relax. Repeat two or three times.

- Raise and tense both shoulders and hold for 10 seconds. Allow them to drop and relax. Repeat three times.

- Rotate each shoulder alternately two or three times – first forwards and then backwards.

- Place the backs of your hands on your lower back. Arch your back by pushing your hips forward and pulling your shoulders back. Hold for 10 seconds and repeat up to three times.

- Stretch both arms out in front of you at shoulder height, palms upright. Bend your forearms back and touch your shoulders with your fingertips. Repeat up to five times.

- Clench your fists tightly for 5 seconds. Stretch your fingers out, then relax them. Repeat up to five times.

10. Switch off!
Switch off from work after hours by turning off your smartphone, iPad or Blackberry and avoiding checking your emails. If you have to bring your work things home with you, put them away so they stay out of sight and out of mind.

De-stress
You can also keep stress in check and neutralise its harmful effects with

relaxation techniques like mindfulness, deep breathing, muscle relaxation and exercise.

Be mindful

Being mindful helps you de-stress because it involves focusing on the here and now, instead of worrying about the future or having regrets about the past. While mindfulness can involve following a particular technique, it doesn't have to – anything you find absorbing will help you to focus on the here and now. For example, try activities like reading, knitting, cooking, drawing, colouring in, walking and playing or watching a sport. However, if you find it hard to stay in the present, try the 'five senses' exercise below to bring you back to the here and now.

'Five senses'

This technique is a great way to practise mindfulness using all of your five senses. Depending on how much time you have to spend, you can do all five steps or just one or two.

1. Notice five things you can **see**.
   Look around you and pick out five things you can see. Focus on each item for a few seconds. What colour is it? What shape is it?

2. Notice four things that you can **feel**.
   Now draw your attention to four things you can feel. For example, your back pressing against the chair you're sitting on, the pressure and warmth of the water if you're having a shower or the breeze on your face if you're outside.

3. Notice three things you can **hear**.
   Now stop and listen – what can you hear? It could be anything from

a bird singing outside to the whirring of traffic from a road nearby.

4. Notice two things you can **smell**.
   Now focus on what you can smell. It could be the perfume or aftershave you're wearing or the smell of pine trees when you're outdoors.

5. Notice one thing you can **taste**.
   Now turn your attention to one thing you can taste. It could be the coffee you've just drunk, something you've just eaten or the taste of a mint in your mouth.

Breathe from your belly

Next time you feel stressed, try taking a deep breath. Deep breathing from your belly is a powerful anxiety-reducing tool because it helps the body switch from the fight-or-flight response of the sympathetic nervous system to the relaxed response of the parasympathetic nervous system. Inhale slowly through your nose allowing your tummy to expand, hold for a few seconds then breathe out through your nostrils while slowly flattening your stomach. Repeat a few times.

Relax your muscles

Tensing your muscles then relaxing them helps you to let go of physical tension and relax. There's evidence that relaxing your body physically can also release psychological tension and stress. Try following these steps to quickly de-stress whenever you feel tense and anxious:

- Slowly inhale, then create tension in your face by clenching your teeth and screwing up your eyes tightly, then relax and breathe out.

- Slowly inhale, then tense your neck and shoulders for a few seconds and then relax, dropping your shoulders and releasing the tension as you exhale.

- Take a deep breath, then clench your fists and tighten the muscles in your arms, hold for a few seconds, then release and breathe out.

- Slowly breathe in, tense the muscles in your buttocks and both of your legs, including the thighs and calves, hold, and then release as you breathe out.

- Finally, slowly inhale clench your toes and tense your feet, hold, then release and exhale.

Say 'yes' to yoga

Yoga can help relieve both the physical and mental effects of stress and calm the gut. Performing the gentle stretching postures and controlled breathing exercises helps you focus on the 'here and now' and release mental and physical tension. In 2016 scientists from the University of Duisburg-Essen, Essen, Germany and the Australian Research Centre in Complementary and Integrative Medicine, Sydney, Australia reviewed six studies involving 273 IBS patients. They found that those who did yoga reported a bigger improvement in their symptoms than those who received conventional treatments.

Exercise away stress

When you exercise, a few things happen in your mind and body that help both prevent and relieve stress:

- The stress hormones adrenaline and cortisol are used up.

- The 'happy' hormone serotonin is released.

- Feel-good endorphins, which relieve stress and boost mood, are produced.

- Your mind is taken off the stresses and strains of daily life.

- Focusing on your chosen activity encourages you to live in the moment.

- Tension is released from your muscles and you breathe more deeply which is relaxing.

- You sleep better because it tires you out physically.

- Your body confidence and self-esteem improve.

- If you go to an exercise class or a gym you benefit from making new friends.

Happy gut tip

You don't need to go to the gym to be active. In the next chapter we look at easy ways to be more active every day.

Get some 'green exercise'

Getting outdoors is known to boost mental and physical well-being. Whether through an active pursuit like walking, gardening or playing an outdoor sport like football, or a passive one like admiring a nice view, getting closer to nature has been shown to lower stress and relieve tension in the muscles.

It's thought that higher levels of negative ions found in places with running water, trees or mountains may play a part. Others think the health boost is due to biophilia – which is the idea that we all have a natural affinity with nature and that our 'disconnection' from it causes stress and mental health problems. In 2016 the World Health Organization (WHO) reported that access to urban green spaces improved mental health by alleviating stress and inducing relaxation.

Sunshine also has an uplifting effect because it boosts vitamin D and serotonin levels. Our skin makes vitamin D on exposure to sunlight. The amount of time you need in the sun to make enough vitamin D varies according to your skin type, the time of day, time of year and where you are in the world. Experts warn against allowing your skin to redden or burn, due to the risk of skin cancer. The general consensus is that spending 10–15 minutes in the UK summer sun without sunscreen several times a week is probably a safe compromise.

Being exposed to soil through gardening is thought to relieve stress and boost mood too – and it's all down to some friendly soil bacteria called *Mycobacterium vaccae*. Once in the gut, like other beneficial bugs, they have an uplifting effect. There are friendly flora in fresh outdoor air too. Exercise has other beneficial effects on gut health – as we shall see in the next chapter.

In a nutshell: why you should dial down stress and how to do it

- Stress can wipe out beneficial gut bacteria and damage the gut.
- Stress can cause weight gain and digestive and sleep problems.
- Dial down stress by boosting your friendly flora, avoiding overload and taking time out to relax.

CHAPTER 10

GET GUT ACTIVE

Regular exercise is important for a healthy digestive system. A lack of exercise can cause constipation because it makes the gut sluggish, so food isn't pushed along the way it should be.

Also, carrying excess pounds around your middle can affect your digestion. The extra weight can put pressure on the stomach, forcing food mixed with stomach acid back up to the gullet – which can cause heartburn. Being overweight can lead to constipation too.

As well as helping you lose weight, as we mentioned in the previous chapter, regular exercise can help cut stress and improve your overall well-being, which in turn can help boost your gut health.

Furthermore, research suggests that regular exercise not only boosts good gut bacteria levels but encourages a wider range of bugs to take up residence in your gut. One study showed that women who exercised three to five times a week had four times as many immunity-boosting *Bifidobacteria* than women who had sedentary lifestyles. It also raises butyrate levels, which calms inflammation and soothes the gut. So being active is vital for a happy, healthy gut.

Remember too that outdoor or 'green' exercise exposes you to the beneficial bacteria in soil and fresh air, which helps to boost mood.

Moderate intensity exercise

Doctors recommend that we do at least 150 minutes of 'moderate intensity physical activity' every week to stay healthy.

According to guidance from the NHS, you're exercising at a **moderate intensity** if you're able to talk, but unable to sing the words to a song.

You may be thinking: 'But I don't have time to exercise for 2½ hours a week.' So wouldn't it be great if you could meet the 2½-hour weekly target without having to find the time to go to the gym or an exercise class?

Fit in fitness

In 2014 Dr Andy Blannin from the University of Birmingham and Dr Chris van Tulleken did a study for the BBC's *Trust Me I'm a Doctor* programme to find out if you can reach the 2½-hour exercise target simply by doing the chores you have to do anyway.

Eight volunteers wore 'activity monitors' while they did everyday household tasks like dusting, mopping, vacuuming, ironing, washing the car, cleaning the windows, mowing the lawn and planting flowers. They found that all of these activities, bar ironing and dusting, met the criteria for moderate intensity exercise.

On average each volunteer spent 109 minutes a week vacuuming and mopping and doing outdoor tasks, suggesting that most of us could easily reach the 2½-hour target no matter how busy our working lives are.

Dr Van Tulleken also pointed out that brisk walking, cycling and carrying a shopping basket instead of using a trolley were also types of moderate intensity exercise. He added that low-intensity exercise like dusting and ironing would still be beneficial, but you would have to do them for longer to get the same health benefits.

Happy gut tip

Dr Blannin's research also showed that how often you exercise is important. Some of the health benefits from moderate activity only last for 12-14 hours afterwards. So he recommends spreading the activities throughout the week, rather than fitting them all into one day.

More sneaky ways to exercise every day

While these all sound like lightweight activities, the effects really do add up if you do them several times each day.

- Get off the bus one stop early.
- Park the car further from work.
- Walk up and down the platform while you wait for your train. You can do the same at the bus stop.
- Take the stairs rather than the lift.
- At work, offer to make a cuppa for your colleagues.
- Go for a short walk on your lunch break.

- Leave your desk and walk around every hour. Go to the photocopier or the water dispenser, pass on a message, make a cuppa or pop to the loo.

- Walk to your local convenience store.

- Walk up and down the escalators rather than standing still.

- Ditch the school run and walk your children to school instead – it'll benefit their health too!

- Take your children to the park or play ball games with them in your garden – again they will benefit from being active too.

- Walk as you talk on your mobile or cordless phone.

- Get up and move around during TV ads, perhaps to make a cuppa or empty the rubbish.

- Wash the car by hand instead of going to the car wash.

- Clean your own windows instead of using a window cleaner.

High intensity interval training (HIIT)

Another shortcut to getting enough exercise to benefit your health when you don't have much time is through high intensity interval training (HIIT), which was shown to be effective on both a BBC *Trust Me I'm a Doctor* programme and a 2012 BBC *Horizon* documentary – *The Truth About Exercise*.

While HIIT might sound difficult, it's quite easy to do. However, because it is a rigorous exercise regime, if you've been inactive for a long time or have any health concerns it's worth getting a check-up with your GP before you start.

1. Warm up

Warm up for 2 minutes before you begin, to help prevent injuries. This could be walking on the spot, joint rotations or some simple stretches.

2. Workout

- Exercise as hard as you can for 60 seconds. You can do any exercise you like as long as it gets you out of breath – for example, running on the spot, skipping, jumping, bouncing on a rebounder or pedalling on an exercise bike.
- Rest for 90 seconds.
- Repeat 60 seconds of exercise then 90 seconds of rest another three times.
- Repeat three times a week.

Happy gut tip

Avoid exercising straight after a meal. If you eat on the move or exercise within 2 hours of eating, you will not only feel sluggish, but the exercise will slow your digestion down and may cause nausea and tummy cramps. Resting after a meal stimulates the vagus nerve, which helps digestion.

In a nutshell: why exercise is good for your gut and how to be more active

- A lack of exercise can cause digestive problems and harmful belly fat.

- Exercise boosts beneficial bugs, helps weight loss and reduces stress.

- You don't need to go to the gym – just fit more activity into your everyday life.

- Outdoor exercise such as gardening can increase numbers of certain friendly gut flora.

PART 4

A GUT-LOVING DAY

CHAPTER 11

BREAKFAST

Breakfast for many of us involves grabbing a slice of toast or a bowl of sugary cereal before dashing off to work. For others a lack of time means leaving the house having eaten nothing at all. But it's generally agreed that breakfast sets us up for the day and helps to prevent snacking on sugary, starchy foods later on in the day, so try to make time to eat something nutritious.

A gut-friendly breakfast should be low in sugar and ideally contain some protein to keep you full for longer, as well as fruit or vegetables for some bug-boosting prebiotics.

Breakfast cereals can provide protein, fibre, vitamins and iron but many contain 10 g of added sugar per serving, so choose unsweetened porridge, Weetabix, shredded wheat or muesli. Remember porridge and muesli are packed with gut-friendly prebiotics. To add natural sweetness and extra prebiotics to your breakfast, top unsweetened cereal with fresh fruit like banana, grated apple, blueberries or strawberries. Yogurt or kefir are also great options if you want a quick, probiotic-boosting breakfast.

The suggestions on the next few pages will help you get your gut-loving day off to a good start.

Happy gut tip

Aim to eat your breakfast, lunch and dinner within a 12-hour window. For example, breakfast at 8 a.m. and dinner no later than 8 p.m. A study at the Salk Institute in California in 2014 found that when mice were restricted to eating a certain amount of food within a set time frame they absorbed fewer calories from it than those who ate the same amount ad lib. They also had a more diverse range of gut bacteria.

Gut-friendly breakfast ideas

- 200 g portion of natural full-fat yogurt with fresh fruit like strawberries, blueberries, raspberries or mango.

- A bowl of porridge with sliced banana or stewed apple, and cinnamon.

- A kefir smoothie made from 100 ml of kefir blended with 150 g of strawberries or blueberries, a small banana and a drizzle of honey. Or try flaxseeds, grated ginger and fresh pineapple or any other combination you fancy.

- A bowl of no-added-sugar muesli topped with a sliced banana and served with milk (dairy or plant-based), or fruit juice.

- Two scrambled eggs, with two handfuls of spinach leaves, on two slices of granary or sourdough toast.

- Two grilled tomatoes with two sliced mushrooms and half a tin of reduced sugar baked beans on two slices of granary or sourdough toast.

Kefir

....

If you can't face eating much first thing in the morning, kefir makes a great, light breakfast drink that's packed with probiotics, protein, vitamins and minerals.

Equipment

2 x 750-ml glass jars – sterilised with boiling water, or washed in dishwasher on hot cycle
1 small plastic sieve

Ingredients

1–2 tbsp of kefir grains   **500 ml** fresh whole milk

Instructions

1. Place kefir grains in one of the glass jars.
2. Add the milk.
3. Gently stir contents, cover jar with a clean cloth or a lid left slightly ajar, and move to a location away from direct sunlight.
4. Allow the mixture to ferment for a minimum of 24 hours.
5. Using the sieve strain the kefir into the other glass jar to remove the kefir grains.
6. You can drink the kefir immediately, or store it in the fridge for up to two weeks.
7. To store the kefir grains return them to the original jar, half fill with milk, seal and place in the fridge until you're ready to start a new batch of kefir.

Happy gut reminder: eat mindfully
Breakfast is the time of day we are most likely to wolf down our food as we rush to leave the house. Remember, eating slowly and chewing your food well is better for your digestion. Try setting your alarm half an hour earlier to give yourself enough time to eat your breakfast without rushing.

Natural yogurt

Home-made yogurt contains more probiotics than shop-bought ones and is easy to make. The powdered milk speeds up the fermentation process and improves the texture, but you can leave it out if you want. Use whole milk and full-fat yogurt to help ensure the good bacteria will survive the acid in your stomach. Makes 1 litre of yogurt.

Equipment
1-litre glass jar – sterilised with boiling water or washed in dishwasher on hot cycle
Digital thermometer (optional)

And/or a **1-litre** Thermos flask – scalded or washed in dishwasher on hot cycle

Ingredients
1 litre whole milk
1 heaped tbsp powdered milk

60 g natural full-fat yogurt

Instructions

1. Put the milk into a saucepan and heat gently until just before it comes to the boil, i.e. just as it starts bubbling at the sides.

2. Take it off the heat and stir in the milk powder.

3. Leave it to cool. When it feels just warm (or 30–40°C if you're using a thermometer) stir in the yogurt. Pour into the jar or Thermos flask and seal with the lid.

4. Put the jar in a warm (not hot) place, such as an airing cupboard, or wrap it in a towel. If you're using a Thermos flask you can leave it anywhere in the kitchen as the yogurt should stay at an ideal temperature for fermentation. Some people store theirs in a microwave overnight, which keeps it warm like a big Thermos flask.

5. Leave for 6–8 hours. If you prefer a more tart flavour you can leave it another hour or two.

6. When the yogurt is ready, store in the fridge for up to five days. If you made the yogurt in a Thermos flask, transfer it into a sterilised glass jar or bowl, cover and place in fridge.

7. Don't forget to leave one or two tablespoons of yogurt to use as a starter culture for your next batch.

Easy muesli

....

This muesli can be made very quickly, because you use a cup to measure the ingredients so there is no weighing involved. The oats, nuts and seeds provide inulin and resistant starch, while the dried fruits provide natural sweetness, vitamins, minerals and fibre.

Ingredients

3 cups oats
1 cup nuts (almonds, hazelnuts, cashew nuts, walnuts or pistachios)
½ cup pumpkin seeds

½ cup sunflower seeds
½ cup raisins
½ cup dried dates or figs, chopped
1 cup dried apricots

Instructions

1. Tip the oats into a large airtight container. Add the nuts, seeds, raisins, dates/figs and dried apricots. Close the container and give it all a good shake to combine the ingredients.
2. Serve with cold milk or, for a probiotic boost, full-fat Greek yogurt.

Smoked salmon and egg muffins
Makes 6

. . . .

These muffins can be served hot or cold and make a great healthy breakfast, or you could eat them with salad for lunch. They can be cooked beforehand and stored in the fridge for a couple of days. The eggs and salmon provide protein and healthy fats that keep you feeling full and less likely to crave sugary food, and repair and soothe your gut lining. The peppers and herbs provide vitamins and antioxidants.

Ingredients

6 eggs
1 red pepper, finely diced

1 tbsp flat leaf parsley or coriander leaves, finely chopped

100 g smoked salmon cut into
small pieces
Olive oil for greasing muffin tray
or you can use a silicone muffin
tray that doesn't need greasing
Sea salt and black pepper,
for seasoning

Instructions

1. Pre-heat oven to 180°C (340°F, fan 160°C, gas mark 4).
2. Place the eggs in a bowl and whisk. Stir in the smoked salmon, red pepper, parsley or coriander. Add a dash of sea salt and black pepper to taste.
3. Bake in the oven for 15 minutes or until they feel firm and turn golden. Serve.

Banana oaty muffins
Makes 6

. . . .

These sugar-free muffins rely on the bananas, cinnamon and raisins for their sweetness. The wholemeal flour provides roughage and stress-busting B vitamins, while the bananas provide prebiotics. If you haven't got time for breakfast first thing, they make a good portable breakfast you can eat later at your desk.

Ingredients

100 g plain wholemeal flour
25 g porridge oats
1 ½ tsp baking powder
½ tsp ground cinnamon
25 g raisins
25 g sunflower spread, melted

25 g light soft brown sugar and mashed
1 egg, beaten **100 ml** skimmed milk
1 medium/large banana, peeled

Instructions

1. Pre-heat oven to 200°C (390°F, fan 180°C, gas mark 6). Line six cups of a muffin tin with paper muffin cases and set aside. Place flour, oatmeal, baking powder and cinnamon in a bowl; mix well. Stir in raisins.

2. In a separate bowl, mix together melted sunflower spread, sugar, egg and milk; add this to flour mixture. Gently fold ingredients together just enough to combine mixture.

3. Gently fold in mashed banana; divide mixture evenly between muffin cups.

4. Bake for about 20 minutes or until risen and golden brown. Serve warm or cold.

Flavour variations

Sultanas, chopped dates, chopped ready-to-eat dried apricots or grated carrot can be used instead of the raisins. You could also replace the cinnamon with grated orange or lemon zest.

These muffins are best eaten freshly baked, but can be kept in an airtight container for 1–2 days.

Spiced winter fruit compote with yogurt
Serves 2

....

This spiced fruit dish makes a warming, immunity-boosting breakfast in the winter. The dried fruits and almonds provide prebiotic fibre, vitamins and minerals, while the yogurt adds probiotics. Greek yogurt is strained, which removes most of the lactose (milk sugar) and whey. This makes it higher in filling protein and lower in sugars than ordinary natural yogurt.

Ingredients

225 g mixed dried fruit (e.g. dried apricots, peaches, pears, apple rings, figs, pitted prunes)
100 ml unsweetened apple juice
100 ml unsweetened orange juice

½ tsp cinnamon
200 ml full-fat Greek yogurt or a plant-based alternative
2 tsp flaked almonds

Instructions

1. Put dried fruit in a large bowl. Pour apple and orange juice into a jug. Add the cinnamon and whisk together. Pour the juice over the fruit and stir well. Cover and chill in fridge for several hours or overnight.
2. To serve cold, remove from fridge and stand at room temperature for about 1 hour before eating.
3. To serve warm, place compote in a microwave-safe container, cover loosely and heat on high until hot (around 2 minutes), pausing after 1 minute to stir. Remove from heat.
4. Share compote between two serving bowls. Top with yogurt, then sprinkle with flaked almonds.

CHAPTER 12

LUNCH

Lunch breaks have all but disappeared, with only one in five of us enjoying a leisurely hour-long lunch and 60 per cent of us eating our lunch at our desks. Little wonder our favourite lunchtime food is the sandwich, which is easy to buy or make, transport and eat.

Unfortunately, shop-bought sandwiches tend be high in fat and sugar and low in protein, fibre and vitamins, so it's far healthier for your gut if you make your own.

Gut-friendly sandwich ideas
- Choose wholemeal bread or pitta to boost your fibre intake.
- If you have problems with gluten, choose more easily digested sourdough bread – see recipe that follows.
- If you're watching your weight, leave out the bread altogether and serve your sandwich filling on little gem lettuce leaves.
- Buy sushi if you're out and about for resistant fibre and protein.
- Choose high-protein fillings like lean meat, tuna, salmon, egg, cheese or prawns to help keep you full and heal your gut.
- Add vegetables or fruit like lettuce, rocket, watercress, cucumber,

beetroot, tomatoes, red onions, avocado or mango for prebiotic fibre, vitamins and minerals.

Sourdough bread

....

Sourdough bread is easier to digest than normal bread because the wild yeast and bacteria in it help to pre-digest the flour and release the nutrients. They also neutralise a substance called phytic acid which is found in grains and can irritate the gut lining. So some people with gluten intolerance find they suffer fewer symptoms from sourdough bread. The lactic acid produced by the bacteria also slows down the rate you digest the glucose so it keeps you full for longer.

Ingredients

300 g strong organic white flour and **150 g** strong organic wholemeal flour, mixed together

300 ml lukewarm water

Starter dough

Instructions

1. Combine 300 g of the organic flour mixture with 300 ml lukewarm water to make a thick paste.
2. Put the paste into a 1-litre glass Kilner jar with the lid slightly open. Leave it in the kitchen at room temperature. If the mixture separates give it a stir.
3. After 3–4 days (depending on how warm your kitchen is) it should be

frothing and smell sour, having picked up the natural airborne yeasts – but discard if it smells unpleasant and start again.

4. Throw or give half the mixture away, then stir in another 150 g of the flour mixture and 150 ml water to make the same quantity as before, but a slightly thicker texture.

5. The next day, take half the mixture to make your first batch of bread. Cover the remaining starter and store in the fridge. Once a week 'feed' it by mixing equal amounts of starter, flour and water. Leave at room temperature for 1–2 hours until slightly bubbly, then re-cover and return to the fridge. When you want to make more bread, simply take it from the fridge and repeat the whole of step 4. Depending how long you've stored and fed it for, you may need to give away or discard more than half the mixture. Leave at room temperature for about 12 hours, or until frothy, before using.

To make 2 loaves of sourdough bread:

Ingredients

500 g strong white organic flour, mixed with **500 g** strong organic wholemeal flour

300 g sourdough starter dough
Approx. **660 ml** water
½ tsp sea salt

Instructions

1. In a large bowl stir the flour mixture, starter and 600 ml water to make a sticky dough. Cover with a clean tea towel. Leave to rest for 20 minutes.

2. Mix the sea salt with three tablespoons of water and combine into the dough. Cover again and leave at room temperature.

3. Leave the dough for about an hour then turn it out onto a work surface. Knead the dough by stretching it out then folding it inwards for about 10 minutes, or until it's smooth and elastic. You'll know it's ready when you can stretch it without it tearing.

4. Cover the dough and leave at room temperature. Every hour or two repeat the stretching and folding.

5. After 6–8 hours pre-heat the oven to 230°C (450°F, fan 210°C, gas mark 8). Meanwhile, halve the dough, shape as desired and place on a baking tray.

6. Bake the loaves for 30–40 minutes until they're golden and sound hollow when tapped on the bottom. Cool on a rack before eating.

Other lunch ideas

- Reduced sugar baked beans on wholemeal, granary or sourdough toast.

- Mashed avocado with halved cherry tomatoes, a dash of olive oil, a squeeze of lemon/lime juice and a handful of fresh coriander served on wholemeal, granary or sourdough toast or rye crispbreads.

- Home-made chunky vegetable soup with added chickpeas or lentils for extra protein and fibre.

- Rye crispbreads or oatcakes with a probiotic-packed cheese such as cottage, gouda, edam, Roquefort, feta or cheddar and tomatoes/sauerkraut (see recipe in **Chapter 14**).

- A selection of vegetable crudités – choose from sticks of carrot, peppers, cucumber, celery, fennel, mushrooms, or whole radishes and sugar snap peas. Serve with home-made hummus or guacamole for extra protein and prebiotic fibre. Find out how to make them in **Chapter 14**.

The leftover lunch

When you cook dinner make an extra portion and store in a lunch box in the fridge or freezer for a quick and easy lunch. Remember that reheated carbohydrates like pasta, rice and potatoes and even bread defrosted from frozen are good sources of the resistant starch that friendly flora love.

If you're tired of sandwiches for lunch, why not ring the changes with one of these tasty, gut-friendly salads?

Tuna and butter bean salad
Serves 2

....

This makes a filling lunch with plenty of fibre to feed your gut bacteria as well as protein to keep you full longer and heal your gut.

Ingredients

200 g can tuna
400 g can butter beans
1 small red onion, thinly sliced
2 large handfuls of rocket
250 g cherry or plum
   tomatoes, halved

2 tbsp olive oil
2 tbsp vinegar
1 tsp wholegrain mustard
Salt and pepper to taste

Instructions

1. Put the sliced red onion into a salad bowl and flake in the tuna. Gently stir in the butter beans and halved cherry or plum tomatoes.
2. Whisk the olive oil, vinegar and wholegrain mustard together. Taste, then add salt and pepper if required. Drizzle the dressing over the salad.
3. Throw in the rocket, gently combine all of the ingredients and serve.

Greek salad
Serves 2

....

This salad captures the flavours of summer while providing beneficial bugs, prebiotics, vitamins A, C and B2 and calcium. The feta also provides filling protein and fats that help you absorb the vitamins.

Ingredients

4 large vine tomatoes, cut into wedges

½ cucumber, roughly chopped

½ red onion, thinly sliced

1 large handful of Kalamata olives (pitted)

1 tsp dried oregano

3 mint leaves, finely chopped

85 g feta cheese, cut into chunks

2 tbsp extra virgin olive oil

1 tbsp red wine vinegar

Instructions

1. Put the tomato wedges into a large salad bowl. Add the onion, cucumber and olives.
2. Spread the feta cheese chunks on top.

3. Sprinkle with the oregano and chopped mint.
4. Drizzle with the extra virgin olive oil and red wine vinegar and serve.

Potato salad
Serves 4

. . . .

This recipe involves chilling the potatoes, so they are full of resistant starch. The full-fat natural yogurt provides probiotics.

Ingredients

1 kg small new potatoes
1 garlic clove, crushed
200 ml full-fat natural yogurt
1 tsp white wine vinegar

3 spring onions, finely sliced
Large handful mint leaves,
   roughly torn
Salt and pepper to taste

Instructions

1. Boil the new potatoes for 15 minutes, or until soft. Drain and cool. Place in the fridge and chill for at least 2 hours, or up to one day.
2. Stir together the crushed garlic, natural yogurt, white wine vinegar and seasoning to make the dressing. This too can be stored in the fridge for up to one day.
3. To serve, stir most of the spring onions and mint into the dressing. Pour it over the potatoes. Combine gently so as not to break up the potatoes. Scatter the remaining spring onions and mint over the salad.

Warm lentil, beetroot and goat's cheese salad
Serves 1

....

Lentils and beetroots contain prebiotic fibre. Beetroot is also rich in betaine, an amino acid thought to boost digestion by increasing stomach acid levels. The goat's cheese provides probiotics.

Ingredients

½ **400 g** can small green lentils, drained and rinsed

2 tsp olive oil

1 tsp wholegrain mustard

½ **bag** mixed salad leaves (about **60 g**)

100 g vacuum-packed cooked beetroot, quartered

50 g soft goat's cheese, sliced

Salt and freshly ground black pepper

Instructions

1. Put the lentils in a saucepan with a teaspoon of olive oil and heat over a low heat until just warmed through. Remove from the heat and stir in the wholegrain mustard.

2. Put the mixed leaves into a serving bowl and put the warm lentils on top. Top with the quartered beetroot and the sliced goat's cheese. Drizzle with the rest of the olive oil and season to taste with the salt and freshly ground black pepper.

Minted pea soup
Serves 2

....

In this soup the peas provide resistant starch, while the mint aids digestion.

Ingredients

1 small onion, chopped
1 large potato (about **225 g**), peeled and diced
500 ml vegetable stock (home-made stocks contain less salt)
225 g peas
2 tbsp fresh mint leaves, finely chopped plus extra leaves to garnish
Freshly ground black pepper, to taste
2 tbsp natural full-fat yogurt or plant-based alternative

Instructions

1. Put the onion, potato and vegetable stock in a saucepan. Bring to the boil, cover with a lid, reduce the heat and simmer until potato is tender (about 15 minutes). Stir every 5 minutes or so.

2. Add the peas, mint and black pepper and stir well. Cover and bring back to the boil. Simmer for 5 minutes.

3. Remove soup from heat. Allow to cool slightly.

4. Using hand-held stick blender, blend soup in pan until smooth. Alternatively, transfer to a blender or food processor and blend until smooth, then return to pan. Reheat over a medium heat until hot.

5. Ladle into soup bowls. Add a swirl of natural yogurt and a sprinkle of chopped mint and serve.

Without the yogurt, this soup can be frozen once cooled for up to three months.

CHAPTER 13

DINNER

When you come home exhausted from a busy day at work, it's all too easy to grab a ready meal or a takeaway, rather than cooking a meal from scratch. But processed foods are usually high in fat, salt and sugar, and low in vitamins and fibre, so they are not good news for your gut health. Home-cooked meals are a much more gut-friendly option. Preparing a gut-healthy evening meal needn't take long, as you'll see from the ideas below.

- Stir-fries only take minutes to prepare and cook. If you're pushed for time you can buy packs of stir-fry vegetables that are ready to throw in a pan and cook.
- Broths and casseroles are easy to prepare and cook. Once they're on the hob, or in the oven, you can do other jobs, or sit and relax. For extra speed, substitute frozen vegetables for fresh.
- Make your own healthier versions of ready meals by cooking extra portions of your favourite dishes and freezing them.

Faster pasta

Roast vegetables such as peppers, tomatoes, onions and courgettes in a little olive oil with garlic, chilli and herbs. Stir in wholewheat pasta that has been pre-cooked, chilled then reheated. Stir in a dash of olive oil to coat the pasta. Add pieces of cooked chicken breast or salmon, or canned tuna for protein. Sprinkle with parmesan shavings for added calcium and probiotics.

Happy gut tip

Cook your rice, pasta or potatoes on a weekend, ready for the week ahead, and freeze. Not only will it save you time every evening, it will also boost your resistant starch intake. Remember, rice should be cooled and chilled or frozen quickly. Store in the fridge for no longer than 24 hours. Reheat only once, to avoid the risk of food poisoning. If frozen, defrost in the microwave or in boiling water, then eat cold or reheat.

Chicken and bone broth
Serves 2

....

This tasty, warming broth contains protein from the chicken meat and gelatine from the chicken bones to soothe and protect your gut lining, while the garlic and vegetables provide prebiotics. This isn't quick to make, so you may want to prepare and cook it at the weekend. You can then freeze it and eat it during the week if you wish.

Ingredients

1 whole chicken
  (organic, if possible)
2 cloves garlic, crushed
2 onions, chopped
2 sticks of celery, chopped

3 carrots, peeled and
  roughly chopped
3 leeks, roughly chopped
2 sprigs fresh rosemary
750 ml water

Instructions

1. Put the chicken into a large pan and cover with the water. Bring to the boil and skim off the scum from the top. Simmer gently for 2 hours, adding more water if needed.

2. Lift the chicken from the pan with a pair of tongs and place on a plate. Remove as much chicken as possible from the carcass. Put the chicken and chicken legs back into the pan. Discard the rest of the chicken.

3. Add all of the vegetables, garlic and herbs to the pot and bring back to the boil. Turn the heat down and simmer for another 2 hours.

4. Remove the chicken leg bones and rosemary sprigs and serve.

Happy gut tip

If you're not keen on chicken broth, you can get the gut-soothing benefits of gelatine by eating jelly – preferably a sugar-free version. Jelly is made from gelatine, which contains the amino acid glycine, which helps to heal and repair the gut lining.

Eat mindfully reminder

Remember to make the time to sit and relax and enjoy your meal. Focus on the taste and texture of your food and chew it well. Avoid leaping up from the table straight after eating. Following these good eating habits will aid your digestion and help you manage your weight.

Salmon and rocket pasta with lemon and basil sauce
Serves 2

The salmon in this pasta recipe gives you gut-soothing protein and omega 3 fats, while the crème fraiche provides probiotics. The basil, rocket and lemon add vitamins and minerals. It's also quick and easy to make – ideal for when you've had a busy day at work and you're too tired to spend hours slaving over a hot stove! Cook the pasta and chill the day before if you can for extra resistant starch.

Ingredients

1 tsp olive oil
2 fresh salmon fillets
200 g pre-cooked and chilled wholewheat pasta
100 g bag of rocket

2 tbsp crème fraiche
Zest of half a lemon
2 tbsp torn basil leaves
½ cup boiling water

Instructions

1. Heat the olive oil in a non-stick pan and cook the salmon over a low-medium heat skin-side down for 5 minutes. Turn the salmon over and cook for a further 4 minutes, until the salmon is cooked through.

2. Remove from pan and leave to cool.

3. Break the salmon up into large chunks, discarding the skin.

4. Add 1–2 tablespoons of water to the pre-cooked pasta and microwave for 2–3 minutes (depending on the power of your microwave) until thoroughly reheated.

5. Drain any remaining water from the reheated pasta. Gently fold in the salmon, crème fraiche, lemon zest, basil and rocket. Stir in some boiling water, a little at a time, until the crème fraiche sauce is the right consistency. Serve immediately.

Crunchy vegetable rice bowl
Serves 2

....

This delicious crunchy vegetable rice bowl can be served alone as a light vegetarian meal, or you can top it with a pan-fried chicken breast, a salmon or sea bass fillet, or a portion of good quality meat, for a more substantial non-vegetarian meal.

The brown rice provides protein, B vitamins, manganese and fibre, while the red pepper and spring onions provide vitamins. The cashew nuts provide protein and gut-soothing healthy fats, as well as iron and calming magnesium. The garlic and celery add prebiotics.

Ingredients

150 g brown basmati rice

5-cm piece fresh root
    ginger, peeled

1 garlic clove

1 red pepper, cut into matchsticks

1 large carrot, cut into matchsticks

2 large spring onions, halved and
    cut into thin strips

½ stick of celery, cut into
    small sticks

4 tbsp raw cashew nuts

2 tbsp light soy sauce

1 tbsp olive oil

3–4 tbsp chopped fresh coriander

Instructions

1. Cook the rice according to the instructions on the pack. To increase the resistant starch, cook the day, or at least a few hours, before. Allow to cool for a few minutes, then cover and refrigerate until ready to use.

Reminder: cooked rice can be stored in a fridge for up to one day.

2. While the rice is cooking, shave the ginger into very thin strips with a vegetable peeler and peel and crush the garlic.

3. Heat a wok until it's really hot, then add the olive oil. As soon as the oil starts smoking, add the ginger shavings, crushed garlic, red pepper, carrot, spring onions, celery and cashew nuts. Keep stirring the vegetables, turning them over every few seconds so they all get the heat from the bottom of the wok. Cook the vegetables until they are softened but still slightly crunchy and the cashews are golden.

4. When the rice is cooked, spoon into a mixing bowl. Toss in the stir-fried vegetables. Add the soy sauce and combine with a fork. Stir in nearly all of the chopped coriander into the rice, still using a fork.

5. Divide between two small bowls, place the chicken or fish on top (if including) then sprinkle with the remaining chopped coriander and serve.

Ricotta, spinach and basil pancakes
Makes 3

....

The egg in these pancakes provides protein, vitamins and gut-soothing fats, while the wholemeal flour gives roughage. The spinach adds prebiotics, vitamins A and K, folic acid and minerals. The ricotta adds gut-friendly bacteria. They're also quick and easy to make.

Ingredients

75 g plain flour (half white,
   half wholemeal)
Pinch of salt
1 egg

200–300 ml milk
1 tbsp basil leaves, finely chopped
Olive oil or rapeseed oil, for frying

For the filling

150 g frozen spinach, defrosted
   with water squeezed out
150 g ricotta cheese

Pinch of grated nutmeg
Salt and freshly ground black
   pepper for seasoning

Instructions

1. To make the pancake batter, put the flour in a bowl. Add the egg, milk, basil and salt. Whisk together until the batter has the consistency of double cream.

2. Heat a little oil in a large frying pan over a medium heat for about 1 minute. Add one ladle of batter and swirl to spread it evenly across the pan.

3. Cook for 1–2 minutes on each side then remove. Repeat to make three pancakes.

4. Meanwhile mix spinach, ricotta and nutmeg in a bowl. Season with salt and freshly ground black pepper.

5. Place pancakes on a clean, flat surface. Share spinach and ricotta filling between pancakes, roll up and serve with salad.

Happy gut reminder: avoid eating too late at night
Remember, eating within a 12-hour window gives your gut a rest overnight, boosts good gut bacteria and helps you manage your weight.

Vegetable chilli with brown rice
Serves 2

....

The vegetables and beans in this chilli provide plenty of prebiotic fibre, vitamins and minerals, while the rice adds B vitamins, protein and flora-friendly fibre.

Ingredients

150 g basmati brown rice, pre-cooked and chilled for extra resistant starch

1 tsp cumin seeds

3 tbsp olive or rapeseed oil

1 small onion, chopped

2 carrots, diced

½ red pepper, seeds removed and chopped

½ yellow pepper, seeds removed and chopped

2 sticks celery, chopped

½ green pepper, seeds removed and chopped

2 x 400 g cans chopped tomatoes

400 g can red kidney beans, drained

200 g can sweetcorn, drained

1–2 red chillies, seeds removed and finely chopped

3 garlic cloves, peeled and roughly chopped

4 tbsp natural full-fat yogurt

4 tbsp fresh coriander
 leaves, chopped

Salt and freshly ground
 black pepper

Instructions

1. Cook the brown rice according to the instructions on the pack. To increase the resistant starch, do this the day, or at least a few hours, before. Allow to cool, cover then refrigerate until needed (up to 24 hours).
2. For the chilli, heat the oil in a large pan. Gently fry the onion over a medium heat until soft, but not brown.
3. Add the carrots, peppers, celery, garlic and chillies and fry for 5 minutes until softened. Pour in the chopped tomatoes and stir well. Bring the mixture to the boil, then turn down the heat and simmer for 15 minutes.
4. Stir in the kidney beans and sweetcorn and continue to simmer until the vegetables are tender. Season to taste with salt and freshly ground black pepper.
5. Add two tablespoons of water to the brown rice then place in a microwave and heat until thoroughly reheated. Stir in the cumin seeds.
6. Share the brown rice between two bowls. Top with the chilli. Drizzle each bowl with a tablespoon of natural yogurt. Scatter a tablespoon of coriander leaves and serve.

Kombucha

....

This fermented tea is rich in beneficial bugs which produce B vitamins during fermentation. It's slightly fizzy, so it makes a healthy alternative to other soft drinks. Try a glass with your evening meal instead of a glass of wine.

Equipment

1.5-litre glass jar (check it can withstand boiling water)

1 muslin cloth

Ingredients

3 green or black teabags

80 g granulated sugar (don't worry – the bacteria digest this!)

900 ml boiling water

Kombucha culture (also called a kombucha 'scoby')

Instructions

1. Put the teabags in the glass jar. Then pour in boiling water almost to the top of the jar. Stir then leave for half an hour. Stir in the sugar until dissolved. Remove the teabags and leave the liquid to cool.

2. Next, add your scoby (which looks a bit like a mushroom) and any liquid that comes with it. Cover the glass jar with the muslin secured with an elastic band or string. Leave it in a place away from direct sunlight and with a steady temperature.

3. Leave the kombucha to ferment. This will take anything from 5 to 18 days. As it ferments the colour will change and it will turn cloudy. Taste it after 5 days. Once it tastes fruity and tart and has a bit of a fizz, it's ready. The longer you leave it, the more sour and less sweet it will be. It's up to you to decide when you think it's ready.

4. When the taste suits you, pour the kombucha through a nylon sieve into a large glass bottle or jug – leaving behind about a quarter of it in

the jar with the scoby. This is what you will use to make your next brew, so store it in the fridge, preferably for just a few days before making another batch.

5. You can flavour your kombucha with fruits, as well as spices and herbs, for extra gut-health benefits. Here are a few ideas to get you started:

- Lemon and ginger – a few squeezes of fresh lemon with freshly grated ginger
- Strawberry and basil – chopped strawberries and fresh torn basil leaves
- Apple and cinnamon – grated apple and dried cinnamon

CHAPTER 14

FERMENTED PICKLES AND GUT-FRIENDLY DIPS

Fermented pickles provide probiotics including various strains of *Lactobacillus*, so they're a great way of getting good bacteria into your gut. Also, the vegetables provide prebiotic fibre for the friendly flora to feed on and flourish.

Equipment: To make each of the fermented vegetable pickles below you'll need two sterilised 500-ml glass jars with screw-tops, or two sterilised 500-ml pickling jars with rubber seals and levers.

Simple sauerkraut

....

Sauerkraut tastes like an acidic coleslaw. It is simple to make, and the home-made version contains far more bacteria than the shop-bought ones, as they tend to be pasteurised which kills off any probiotics. You only need a tablespoon a day to benefit. Try adding it to salads and sandwiches or on crackers with goat's cheese.

Ingredients

1 large cabbage (any type will work – including red cabbage), cut into 1-cm thick slices

1 tbsp of sea salt
1 tbsp of caraway seeds
1 tbsp of peppercorns

Instructions

1. Place the sliced cabbage in a clean bowl.
2. Mix in the sea salt, caraway seeds and peppercorns with your hands.
3. Keep pummelling the cabbage with your hands (or you can use a pestle or the end of a rolling pin) for 10–20 minutes, until the cabbage has released a fair amount of liquid.
4. Transfer the mixture into the sterilised jars, making sure the cabbage is covered with the liquid, but leave a 2-cm gap at the top to allow for the mixture to froth and fizz.
5. Store at room temperature and out of direct sunlight for three days to three weeks.
6. Open the jar every day for the first three days to release any carbon dioxide (known as 'burping') and check the cabbage is still covered in brine, pushing it down if necessary.
7. The longer you leave the cabbage fermenting, the stronger the flavour, so taste it regularly with a clean spoon. Once you're happy with the flavour, store it in the fridge where it will keep for several months.

Food safety

With all of these fermented vegetable pickle recipes, make sure you practise good hygiene to avoid introducing potentially harmful bacteria. All equipment, including the glass jars, should be put through the hot cycle in the dishwasher – or washed, then sterilised with boiling water, before you start. Also, don't forget to wash your hands thoroughly with hot water and soap or handwash.

Kimchi

....

Kimchi is a traditional Korean spicy pickle made with fermented vegetables. It's quite salty and acidic and goes well with rice dishes.

Ingredients
For the fermented vegetables
1 Chinese cabbage
1 tbsp sea salt
8 radishes, coarsely grated

2 carrots, coarsely grated
4 spring onions, finely shredded

For the kimchi paste
3 garlic cloves, crushed
2½-cm piece ginger, grated
2 tbsp Thai fish sauce or soy sauce
2 tbsp chilli paste

1 tsp caster sugar
3 tbsp rice vinegar or organic live
apple cider vinegar

Instructions

1. Slice cabbage into 2.5-cm strips. Put into a bowl and mix with the sea salt. Put to one side for 1 hour.
2. Meanwhile make the kimchi paste. Blend the garlic, ginger, Thai fish sauce or soy sauce, chilli paste, sugar and rice vinegar or apple cider vinegar together in a bowl.
3. Wash the cabbage under cold running water, drain and dry thoroughly.
4. Transfer to a large sterilised bowl and toss with the kimchi paste, radishes, carrots and spring onions.
5. Put into sterilised glass jars. Seal and leave to ferment at room temperature.
6. During the first 3–4 days you'll need to remove the jar lid to allow the fermentation gases to escape.
7. The kimchi should be ready in 10–14 days, when the vegetables have softened. It will then need to be stored in the fridge, where it'll keep for a few weeks.

Fermented beetroot

....

Fermented beetroots retain more of their nutrients than boiled beetroots pickled in vinegar, and offer the added benefit of bug-boosting probiotics.

Ingredients

400 g raw beetroot, peeled and cut into large matchsticks

2 tbsp sea salt
500 ml water

Instructions

1. Put the beetroot matchsticks into the sterilised jars.
2. Add the salt to the water and stir until dissolved. Pour over the beetroot, making sure it's completely submerged.
3. Close the jar lids and keep at room temperature, out of bright sunlight. Open the lids every couple of days to 'burp' the mixture.
4. Start tasting the beetroot after three days to check how sour it is. Leave it fermenting until you're happy with the taste. Then store in the fridge.

Tip: Serve with feta cheese and rye crispbreads for a tasty probiotic lunch.

Fermented garlicky carrots

....

The garlic in these fermented carrots packs a real punch and adds extra prebiotics to help feed the friendly flora from fermentation.

Ingredients
400 g carrots
4 garlic cloves, peeled

2 tbsp sea salt
500 ml water

Instructions

1. Peel the carrots and cut them into sticks by quartering them. For longer carrots cut them in half again.
2. Share the garlic cloves between the two sterilised glass jars.
3. Place the carrot sticks into the jars upright and on top of the garlic.

Pack them tightly, but make sure there's enough room for the brine to circulate around them.

4. Stir the salt into the water until it's dissolved. Pour over the carrot sticks, making sure they're completely covered.

5. Secure the lids tightly. Store the jars at room temperature out of direct sunlight. 'Burp' the mixture every couple of days.

6. After seven days, start tasting the carrots. As soon as you like the taste – which can take up to two weeks – store in the fridge.

Alternative flavour combinations: Replace the garlic with a sprig of any herb of your choice, e.g. rosemary or thyme. Or add a slice of fresh peeled ginger root.

Home-made hummus

....

Hummus is made with chickpeas, which are a great source of protein and prebiotics. This hummus is delicious served with strips of wholemeal pitta bread and raw carrot, cucumber and pepper sticks.

Ingredients

200 g can chickpeas
2 tbsp lemon juice
2 garlic cloves, crushed
1 tsp ground cumin
Pinch of salt

1 tbsp tahini (sesame seed paste)
4 tbsp water
2 tbsp extra virgin olive oil
1 tsp paprika

Instructions

1. Drain the chickpeas and rinse.
2. Mix together the chickpeas, lemon juice, olive oil, garlic, cumin, salt, tahini and water, then blend to a creamy texture.
3. Taste the mixture then add more lemon juice, garlic, cumin or salt if needed.
4. Sprinkle with paprika and serve. You can vary the flavour by making the hummus as above and then choosing any of the additional ingredients below:

   - **Coriander hummus:** Blend in two tablespoons of fresh chopped coriander to help beat the bloat.

   - **Beetroot hummus:** Blend in two peeled cooked beetroots for extra fibre. You can use vacuum-packed beetroot if you like.

   - **Basil and parmesan hummus:** Blend in two tablespoons of anti-inflammatory and antibacterial basil leaves. Stir in two tablespoons of grated parmesan for gut-friendly microbes.

   - **Red pepper hummus:** Char one large halved and deseeded red pepper. Cut into pieces, then blend in. Red peppers are green peppers that have ripened, making them easier to digest.

Guacamole

....

The avocados in this recipe give you gut-soothing, anti-inflammatory monounsaturated fats and phytosterols, as well as fibre and vitamin C.

Ingredients

2 large, ripe avocados
1 tbsp extra virgin olive oil
1 garlic clove, crushed or
    finely chopped
Juice of 1 lime

Sea salt and black pepper
Finely chopped green chilli,
    tomato, red onion and
    coriander (optional)

Instructions

1. Either blend all the ingredients together or, for a more chunky texture, mash the ingredients together in a bowl.
2. Stir in lime juice, oil and seasoning to taste.

Happy gut tip

If your avocados are too hard, wrap them in some newspaper. Avocados produce a gas called ethylene which helps ripen them. Wrapping them up traps the ethylene and speeds up the process. Or store them in a fruit bowl containing bananas, which also give off ethylene. Check every few hours. A ripe avocado should be dark green and feel slightly squidgy.

FINAL THOUGHTS

If you want to improve your physical and mental health, take good care of your gut and you'll soon reap the rewards. If you start following the gut-friendly diet and lifestyle tips in this book today, you'll quickly see big improvements in your health and well-being.

As this book has shown you, making your gut happy doesn't have to be complicated. Simply enjoy a healthy, varied diet. Eat plenty of good quality protein foods, fruit, vegetables, wholegrains, dairy foods, nuts and seeds and include some fermented foods. Avoid processed starchy and sugary foods and try to keep a lid on stress. Enjoy tea, coffee, wine and dark chocolate in moderation. Avoid taking unnecessary medication. Get active every day – preferably outdoors. Follow good sleep habits, relax and enjoy life with your family and friends.

I hope I've inspired you to try making your own fermented foods and to cook more gut-friendly meals. The information, advice and tips in this book should help you on your way towards a happier gut. Quite simply, if you look after your friendly flora, they'll look after you!

JARGON BUSTER

Below are the meanings of some of the words linked to gut health that are used in this book and that you may come across in other books and websites on the subject.

Anti-inflammatory – describes a substance that reduces swelling, pain and inflammation.

Anus – the opening at the end of the digestive system from which faeces (waste) leave the body.

Bile – a yellow fluid produced by the liver that is stored in the **gall bladder** and released to aid the digestion of fats.

Biome – a shorthand for **microbiome**.

Butyrate – a short-chain fatty acid (SCFA) produced by gut bacteria that nourishes the gut lining.

Carminative – describes a substance that prevents gas forming in the gut, or eases its passing.

Chyme – partially digested food that has been mixed with acids in the stomach.

Cortisol – stress hormone produced by the adrenal glands.

Digestion – the breaking down of food into smaller pieces to enable the body to absorb the nutrients in it.

Duodenum – the first part of the small intestine.

Dysbiosis – this is where the healthy balance between good and bad bacteria is disrupted and harmful microbes take hold, causing a range of health problems.

Enteric nervous system – the nervous system in the gut (the 'gut-brain') that sends and receives messages to and from the brain via the **vagus nerve**.

Enzyme – a protein produced in the body to speed up processes like digestion.

Epiglottis – the flap at the back of the tongue that prevents chewed food from going down the windpipe to the lungs. When you swallow, your epiglottis automatically closes. When you breathe, it opens, allowing air to go in and out of the windpipe.

Flora (gut flora) – tiny bacteria that inhabit your gut and help to digest your food. They also produce vitamins, minerals and hormones vital to good health.

Gall bladder – a small, sac-like organ that stores bile and releases it into the small intestine.

Gastric – literally means 'of the stomach'.

Gastric juice – liquid made in the stomach that contains hydrochloric acid and enzymes to break down food.

Gastroenterology – the study of the digestive system.

Gastrointestinal – linked to, or referring to, the stomach and intestines.

Glycaemic index – a ranking of foods according to the effect they have on blood sugar levels.

Ileum – the last part of the small intestine.

IBS – irritable bowel syndrome.

Jejunum – the middle part of the small intestine.

Laxative – something that stimulates a bowel movement.

Liver – a large organ in front of and just above the stomach; it filters toxins from the blood and makes bile to digest fats.

Malfermentation – abnormal fermentation of food by 'bad' bacteria, which results in the release of toxic waste and gases.

Melatonin – hormone made by the pineal gland in the brain which regulates sleep.

Microbiome – a collection of **microbiota** (see below), for example, the gut microbiome that lives in our gut. Also used to describe the genetic information of microbiota.

Microbiota – microbes (bacteria) that live in the body (e.g. the gut) or on the skin.

Oesophagus – the long tube that uses rhythmic muscle movements (**peristalsis**) to push food from the throat down into the stomach.

Pancreas – a gland just below the stomach and above the intestines that makes enzymes to help digestion. It also makes the hormone insulin and releases it into the bloodstream, where it regulates the levels of glucose (sugar) in the blood.

Peristalsis – involuntary rhythmic muscle movements that push food along the oesophagus from the throat down into the stomach.

Polyphenols – natural plant chemicals that boost beneficial bacteria in the gut.

Prebiotics – natural indigestible starches that feed and encourage the growth of existing 'good' bacteria in the gut.

Probiotics – literally means 'for life'. Beneficial bacteria found in foods, such as natural yogurt, which are thought to aid digestion.

Rectum – the lower part of the large intestine, where faeces are stored before they are expelled from the body.

Saliva – fluid produced by **salivary glands** and containing enzymes that break down carbohydrates (starch) into smaller molecules.

Salivary glands – glands located in the mouth that produce saliva.

Serotonin – a chemical involved in various bodily functions, including mood, appetite, sleep and sensory perception.

Short-chain fatty acids (SCFAs) – fats such as **butyrate**, produced by gut bacteria when they break down fibre in the gut.

Stomach – a sack-like, muscular organ that is joined to the oesophagus, where both chemical and physical digestion happens.

Vagus nerve – nerve that extends from the brain to the gut and helps manage digestion, including telling the stomach muscles to contract and push food into the small intestine.

Villi – finger-like protrusions in the small intestine that help nutrient absorption.

RESOURCES

If you'd like to learn more about the topics we've covered in this book, you may find the following lists of books and websites helpful.

Books

Bassford, Katherine **Oh Sugar! How to Satisfy Your Sweet Tooth Naturally for a Happy, Healthy Lifestyle** (2015, Summersdale) – a useful guide to cutting down on sugar in your diet, which is helpful when aiming to improve your gut health.

Enders, Giulia **Gut: The Inside Story of Our Body's Most Under-rated Organ** (2015, Scribe) – a witty and informative guide to the gut and gut bacteria and the vital role they play in our health.

Green, Wendy **IBS: A Self-Help Guide to Feeling Better** (2016, Summersdale) – a practical guide to managing irritable bowel syndrome (IBS).

Knight, Rob **Follow Your Gut: The Enormous Impact of Tiny Microbes** (2015, Simon & Schuster) – a fascinating explanation of what the gut biome is and does.

Sonnenburg, Justin and Erica **Gut Reactions: How Healthy Insides Can Improve Your Weight, Mood and Well-Being** (2017, Corgi) – explains the role gut bacteria play in your health and contains recipes, meal plans and day-to-day advice.

Websites

www.coeliac.org.uk – expert advice to help people with coeliac disease manage their condition.

www.corecharity.org.uk – a gut health charity that offers evidence-based information on a wide range of digestive disorders.

www.loveyourgut.com – lifestyle and diet tips and gut-friendly recipes to improve gut health.

www.tummytrouble.co.uk – provides information on tummy aches and pains including causes, symptoms and relief.

PRODUCTS

The emphasis in this book is on improving your gut health by changing your diet and lifestyle, rather than by taking supplements. But if you've recently taken a course of antibiotics or non-steroidal anti-inflammatory drugs (NSAIDs) such as aspirin or ibuprofen, or had a gut infection, you may benefit from taking probiotics for a month or two.

Probiotics

The probiotics listed below contain species and strains that clinical research suggests improve digestive and other health issues.

OpticBac – www.optibacprobiotics.co.uk
ProVen – www.provenprobiotics.co.uk

Also, if you suffer from wind and bloating, as well as using herbs and spices like peppermint and ginger you may want to try activated charcoal, which has been clinically proven to relieve these complaints.

Medicinal charcoal

Made from coconut shells. Available in biscuit, capsule, tablet and powder form. You can find out more about the health benefits of charcoal and how it works on the website below.

J.L. Bragg's Medicinal Charcoal – www.charcoal.uk.com

ACKNOWLEDGEMENTS

I'd like to thank Claire Plimmer, editorial director at Summersdale, for giving me the opportunity to write a title on such a fascinating topic. I'm also grateful to Robert Drew and Liz Bourne for their very helpful editorial input. I'd also like to thank my husband Gordon for being supportive and never complaining about the nights I spent at the computer working on this book!

ABOUT THE AUTHOR

Wendy Green is the author of over a dozen books about health and well-being. In 2000 she gained a BSc first-class honours degree in Health Studies. During her degree she studied health from all angles – including the psychological, biological, nutritional, environmental and social factors that affect our well-being. As a result, all of her books cover their topic holistically, with suggestions on how to overcome health issues through diet, exercise, managing stress and following good sleep habits. She believes that adopting a healthier lifestyle needn't involve following a restrictive diet or a punishing exercise regime, but that making small but long-term tweaks to your diet and lifestyle can lead to huge improvements in your health. She has run a health project for the Deaf community for more than ten years.

IBS

A self-help guide to feeling better

Wendy Green

Foreword by Dr Nick Read,
chair of The IBS Network

IBS

A self-help guide to feeling better

Wendy Green

£8.99
Paperback
ISBN: 978-1-84953-807-7

In this easy-to-follow book, Wendy Green explains how food intolerances, gut infections and bacterial imbalance, and stress and hormones contribute to IBS, and offers practical advice and a holistic approach to help you deal with the symptoms, including simple dietary and lifestyle changes, and DIY complementary therapies. Find out 50 things you can do today to help you cope with IBS, including:

- Identify your IBS triggers and learn how to manage them
- Choose beneficial foods and supplements
- Manage stress and relax to reduce flare-ups
- Discover practical tips for living with IBS
- Adopt preventative strategies
- Find helpful organisations and products

Have you enjoyed this book?
If so, why not write a review on your favourite website?

If you're interested in finding out more about our books,
find us on Facebook at **Summersdale Publishers** and
follow us on Twitter at **@Summersdale**.

Thanks very much for buying this Summersdale book.

www.summersdale.com